COMMUNICATING
HEALTH
STRATEGIES FOR HEALTH PROMOTION

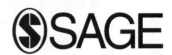

2ND EDITION

COMMUNICATING HEALTH

STRATEGIES FOR HEALTH PROMOTION

EDITED BY **NOVA CORCORAN**

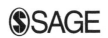

Los Angeles | London | New Delhi
Singapore | Washington DC

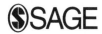

SAGE

Los Angeles | London | New Delhi
Singapore | Washington DC

SAGE Publications Ltd
1 Oliver's Yard
55 City Road
London EC1Y 1SP

SAGE Publications Inc.
2455 Teller Road
Thousand Oaks, California 91320

SAGE Publications India Pvt Ltd
B 1/I 1 Mohan Cooperative Industrial Area
Mathura Road
New Delhi 110 044

SAGE Publications Asia-Pacific Pte Ltd
3 Church Street
#10-04 Samsung Hub
Singapore 049483

Editor: Alice Oven
Assistant editor: Emma Milman
Production editor: Katie Forsythe
Copyeditor: Jane Fricker
Proofreader: Bryan Campbell
Marketing manager: Tamara Navaratnam
Cover design: Wendy Scott
Typeset by: C&M Digitals (P) Ltd, Chennai, India
Printed by MPG Printgroup, UK

Editorial supervision, Introduction, Chapter 1, Chapter 4,
Chapter 5, Chapter 9 © Nova Corcoran 2013
Chapter 2 © Nova Corcoran and Sue Corcoran 2013
Chapter 3 © Calvin Moorley, Barbara Goodfellow and
Nova Corcoran 2013
Chapter 6 © Nova Corcoran, Anthony Bone and
Claire Everett 2013
Chapter 7 © Nova Corcoran and John Garlick 2013
Chapter 8 © Sue Corcoran 2013

First edition published 2007. Reprinted in 2008 and twice in 2010.
This edition first published 2013

Library of Congress Control Number: 2012942960

British Library Cataloguing in Publication Data

A catalogue record for this book is available from
the British Library

ISBN 978-1-4462-5232-1
ISBN 978-1-4462-5233-8 (pbk)

CONTENTS

LIST OF FIGURES

ABOUT THE EDITOR

Nova Corcoran works as a Senior Lecturer in Public Health at the University of Glamorgan where she is the award leader for the MSc Public Health. She is the author and editor of two textbooks 'Communicating health: Strategies for health promotion' and 'Working on health communication'. She previously held the post of Senior Lecturer in Health Promotion and Public Health at the University of East London for 10 years. Prior to that she worked in a variety of health promotion roles including the role of Addiction Prevention Practitioner at St Georges Hospital Medical School, and as a Health Promotion Officer and Stop Smoking Development Coordinator for Cornwall and the Isles of Scilly Health Authority. She has a strong background in health promotion work, in particular the planning, design and delivery of health campaigns and programmes. Her research interests are centred on communication strategies and methods including mass media, social marketing, behaviour change and international health issues.

LIST OF CONTRIBUTORS

Anthony Bone works as a Principal Lecturer in Health Studies at the University of East London. He has a background in higher education, and an interest in health and social policy.

Sue Corcoran is an Assistant Director of Nursing at the Royal Cornwall Hospitals Trust. She has worked in a variety of settings in nursing and midwifery in primary and acute care, higher education and senior NHS management. She has retired since the first edition of this textbook.

Claire Everett is a nutrition and health promotion consultant. She currently works as a Commissioning Manager for the Food for Life Partnership and has a teaching and research interest in food-related areas.

John Garlick is a Principal Lecturer in Health Service Management at the University of East London. He has worked extensively on health care policy development and on service delivery in central government and at local level in North East London. He has retired since the first edition of this textbook.

Barbara Goodfellow works as a Senior Lecturer in Medical Sociology at the University of East London. She has a nursing background and her particular interests are inequalities in health, especially those relating to culture, gender and old age. She has retired since the first edition of this textbook.

Calvin Moorley is a Senior Lecturer in Health Promotion and Health Studies at the University of East London. His main interests are in how culture influences health and the meaning of illness. He comes from a nursing background, with a critical and primary care specialism.

EDITOR'S ACKNOWLEDGEMENTS

Thank you to all my students and colleagues past and present from the University of East London and the University of Glamorgan for making my job worthwhile. This edition is dedicated to Ben, Ostyn and Huxley.

Nova Corcoran

INTRODUCTION TO THE SECOND EDITION

NOVA CORCORAN

There is likely no better time to be working in the area of health communications. Whether studying it or applying it, we are operating in a time that will likely be looked upon as a 'game changer' period in history. (Hesse et al., 2010: S5)

Health communication is at the forefront of any effort to promote health or prevent ill health and health practitioners who engage in health communication through health promotion or public health practice are part of this arena.

Health promotion is a 'dynamic, planned and measurable process' (CCP, 2003) and is used to prevent morbidity and mortality and to promote a notion of holistic health and wellbeing. Communication is at the forefront of the achievement of health promotion objectives. It is at the centre of how human beings are defined and our way of exchanging information with others (Rimal and Lapinski, 2009). Globally health communication is recognised as a huge part of the drive to improve health and reduce inequalities in health. The US Healthy People objectives for 2010 have a whole chapter on 'health communication and health information technology' to achieve 'Healthy People Objectives for 2020' (US Department of Health and Human Services, 2010) illustrating its importance as a vehicle in health care, public health and the way society views health. Low income countries such as Liberia are using billboards to communicate to the population a range of health and citizenship messages to try and encourage widespread changes in societal and cultural norms, values, beliefs and practices (Humphrys, 2012). In the UK the main government campaign to encourage changes in lifestyles centres around a wide scale mass media social marketing campaign – Change4Life (see www.change4life.com). The future of health communication truly is growing and changing to adapt to population and country needs at a fast pace.

Health practitioners frequently engage in efforts to promote health using a variety of communication means and there is a general dependence in health promotion for using campaigns as a primary strategy for public health interventions (Kreps and Maibach, 2008). This trend is set to increase with the rise of information technology (IT) use and applications that engage populations in the dialogue and management of their own health.

While more health care providers now understand that communication is a central social process in the provision of health care delivery and the promotion of public health, many do not always recognise that effective communication is a complex and fragile human process that demands strategic design, careful monitoring and responsive adaptation (Kreps and Neuhauser, 2010). It is also a 'symbolic exchange of shared meaning' (Rimal and Lapinski, 2009: 247) which suggests there is a process of transmitting a message and factors that influence this process.

Communication in health promotion is not a simple linear process of providing information for immediate benefit – an assumption that has frequently been made (Lee and Garvin, 2003). Assuming that communication is a linear process implies that it is a one-way information flow where a message from one source automatically translates to a behaviour change in the receiver. Health practitioners over time have come to realise that good communication in health is actually the movement towards two-way communication. Lee and Garvin (2003) refer to this as a move away from 'monologue' to 'dialogue'; in other words, moving from information transfer (a one-sided approach) to information exchange (a multi-way approach) and the concurrent reflection in health – the move from individual health education to holistic health promotion, a view supported by Thackeray and Neiger (2009).

Daily there are new challenges to (and in) the field of health promotion. The global world of health is changing with the increase of so-called lifestyle-related diseases such as cancers and coronary heart disease and the spread of global diseases such as H1N1 (swine flu) which involve communication across a global environment. This can often be in situations where the need for health promotion outstretches budgets and resources. One premise underpinning health promotion is that all practitioners have good communication skills to enable them to promote health through the design, planning, implementation and evaluation of programmes, campaigns or policies. Changing behaviour is complex, as Caprio et al. (2008) note the public health approach to obesity will need to take into account ethnicity, culture, socioeconomic status, the influences on the child and family such as economics and community resources, geography, built environments, available food, media messages and settings. Practitioners therefore need to develop comprehensive plans and frameworks that take into consideration this extensive range of factors. Noar (2006, 2012) notes that reviews of the communication literature indicate that a range of health communication campaigns continue to fail to adhere to principles of effective campaign design. *Communicating Health: Strategies for health promotion* aims to consider the wide range of influences impacting on health communication and the design of health campaigns to enable practitioners to utilise principles and practice to ensure effectiveness in their work.

The second edition of *Communicating Health: Strategies for health promotion* aims to bring together health promotion and health communication by fusing the link between theory and practice as before, but this time with an updated focus on current issues and practice. It has been a number of years since the original publication of the book and much has changed in campaign practice with the evolution of IT, new mass media campaigns, social marketing techniques and the constantly evolving nature of health communication. *Communicating Health: Strategies for health promotion* aims to focus on these new additions to health communication theory and practice through the provision of new evidence, chapter sub-headings, case studies and activities. Using the same philosophy as the first edition, this updated textbook seeks to try and fill this 'communication gap' in the literature; its premise is that there is little use having a detailed theoretical knowledge base but few skills to implement this knowledge into practice. Likewise, there is little use having the practical skills without the theoretical rationale. If health practitioners continue to work without this fusing of theory and practice, there is a danger of practice becoming at best ineffective, at worst health damaging.

Communicating Health: Strategies for health promotion retains a strong academic focus, allowing practitioners to gain practical theoretical knowledge using a mixture of activities and case studies. It is aimed at the wide audience in the health promotion nexus. Health promotion is a multidisciplinary field attracting practitioners from a range of areas. This includes the overarching fields of health promotion, health education and public health; for example, practitioners in environmental health, communities, schools, hospitals, health centres, and workplaces can all be engaged in health promotion work. This book is also aimed at those who are studying to become health practitioners from the range of disciplines that make up health promotion, including health studies, public health, nursing and other professions allied to medicine.

The text is presented in nine chapters. It commences with content on theoretical models and target groups and logically progresses through key topics to conclude with a chapter on evaluation. The chapters aim to take into account the range of areas that practitioners will encounter when planning, delivering and evaluating programmes, policies and campaigns. Each chapter has a number of activities. The activity discussions are found at the back of the book and are designed to give the reader examples of model answers for these activities. There is also a glossary at the end of the book, and all terms have been highlighted in the text at their first appearance The symbol >> also appears in the margin.

Chapter 1 examines the theories and models that are used in communicating health promotion messages. This chapter provides an overview of both stage-step and cognitive theories. These theories are critiqued and applied to practical situations in a variety of different contexts. Readers are encouraged to explore the theoretical frameworks and apply these to case studies and activities.

Chapter 2 explores the social and psychological factors that are associated with target groups when planning communication campaigns. This is an area that is often overlooked in planning community strategies. This chapter seeks to highlight factors that a health practitioner should be aware of when pre-planning communication campaigns.

Chapter 3 engages with the social and cultural aspects of target groups, drawing on three hard-to-reach groups. These are different cultural groups, people living with a disability and older people. This chapter considers ways to communicate with these groups, taking into account their diversity.

Chapter 4 highlights the role of mass media in health communication, and identifies current uses of mass media. Topics include examining the role of visual and print media, utilising the media for free, branding, message design and social marketing principles. This chapter seeks to enable practitioners to think critically about mass media and consider ways they can use mass media in their work more effectively.

Chapter 5 explores information technology (IT), including current use and future application to health. The role of the Internet, mobile phones and other multi-media IT in health is critiqued. Problems linked to IT in health and ways to overcome these are explored. Other issues that are covered include website design, tailoring information and Internet advocacy.

Chapter 6 examines the settings-based approach from a non-traditional perspective. Frequently, health practitioners will be working in settings to deliver health promotion work. This chapter explores the settings approach, using personal care locations (barbers, beauty salons), places of worship, universities and convenience stores. These settings, which deviate from the usual settings focus, help to demonstrate the versatility of settings for health communication work.

Chapter 7 examines evidence-based practice with the premise that it is essential to the design of health promotion work. This chapter focuses on how a practitioner can use the evidence base in their work, including in the replication and location of appropriate interventions.

Chapter 8 analyses the role of evaluation in health communication. This chapter examines the rationale for evaluation of heath promotion. It considers strategies and methods of evaluation that can be used to illustrate effectiveness of work and the achievement of campaign goals.

Chapter 9 explores 10 different health promotion campaigns that use a variety of strategies and methods to achieve their aims. This is designed to be read after the other chapters when readers are in a position to consider what they have learnt from the textbook and how this can be applied to practice. Website links are provided for all campaigns so readers can explore these campaigns for themselves.

On a last note, much of the research for this book has come from journals and health promotion organisations in the UK and worldwide, drawing on areas that are being constantly updated (for example, IT) where reliance on current information is essential. It is hoped that the second edition of *Communicating Health: Strategies for health promotion* will open the debate around communication in the design of programmes, campaigns and policies to promote health, and thus move closer to reaching fundamental health promotion goals of achieving health for all.

1

THEORIES AND MODELS
NOVA CORCORAN

Learning objectives:

- Define the term 'communication' and identify components of the communication process in a health promotion context.
- Explore communication theory in relation to health promotion practice.
- Apply theoretical models of health promotion to the health promotion and health education setting.

Communication has an essential role in any action that aims to improve and promote health. New models of communication recognise that the communication process involves a multi-way interaction between the sender and receiver of health messages. This chapter will define the communication process and consider four behaviour change models that can be applied in successful campaign and communication design. This includes emphasis on how communication is disseminated through populations as well as influential factors in the communication process. This chapter seeks to bridge the theory to practice gap and emphasises the application of theoretical models to practice.

COMMUNICATION DEFINED

Communication is a transactional process and in a health context it is an important part of health promotion work. It is vital in the achievement of healthy individuals and populations and contributes to the reduction in inequalities. Health communication is understood as 'an enabler of individual and social levels change to achieve established development goals including health' (Suresh, 2011:276).

>> The communication transaction is one of sharing information using a set of common rules (Northouse and Northouse, 1998). In *health promotion* communication is a process that is essential in the achievement of health outcomes. Communication is usually a process that comes to fruition when the audience has achieved, acted on or responded to messages that ultimately aim to increase health goals.

COMPONENTS OF COMMUNICATION

>> Historically the basic representative *model* of communication was usually conceptualised as a one-way flow process consisting of a sender, message and receiver. More recent work in the area of communication added fourth and fifth variables: complete understanding by that receiver and feedback to the communicator. These last two variables hold importance to health communication as they imply two-way communication, enabling a move away from the traditional concept of one-way communication towards multi-way communication. Communication is a cyclic process involving a series of actions, thus a modified model can be represented as circular (see Figure 1.1).

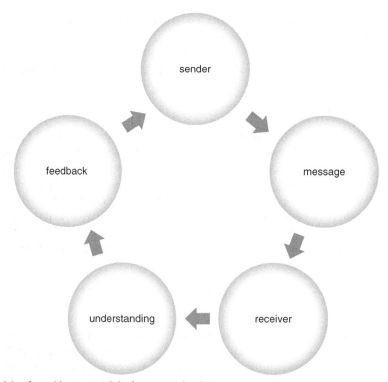

Figure 1.1 A multi-way model of communication

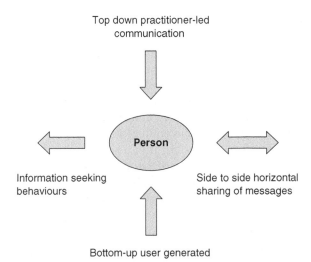

Figure 1.2 A new model of communication, adapted from Thackeray and Neiger (2009)

The most recent developments in health communication reflect the evolving notion that the health communication process is multidirectional as the general population actively seek information from the immediate, accessible formats available to them, for example from the Internet. This has created a model of communication that is no longer an expert-driven top-down model of communication, but a non-hierarchical, horizontal form of communication. Thackeray and Neiger (2009) also concur with this idea and suggest a communication model which emphasises this bottom-up and horizontal approach. This model is represented in Figure 1.2.

This model assumes that communication can be expert-generated from both the top down but also from the bottom up, and therefore user-generated as well as side-to-side sharing (horizontal). It is suggested that effective health communication must involve an active collaborative transaction between the sender and receiver (Kreps and Neuhauser, 2010). This view emphasises that in order for a change to occur, i.e. in a health behaviour, the receiver must take more of a proactive part in the communication process instead of passively receiving messages.

FACTORS INFLUENCING COMMUNICATION

The multidimensional and dynamic nature of communication means that transactions contain other aspects that influence communication. Watzlawick et al. (1967) break communication down into 'content' and 'relationship'. The 'content' includes the message, the words and the information transmitted. The 'relationship' consists of the dynamics between those involved in the communication transaction – the communicator(s). This breakdown has the advantage of identifying the content and the relationship between the sender and receiver separately. In *Communicating Health: Strategies for health promotion* the main sender is the health practitioner and the receiver is the intended audience (who will be discussed in more detail in Chapter 2). Traditionally the relationship between the sender and receiver is defined as horizontal, but as the main focus of this textbook is for the practitioner to develop skills in communication the sender is essentially going to be a health practitioner. The content aspect is currently of considerable interest in this chapter.

The content of a message contains verbal and non-verbal communication. Verbal communication is the words, sentences and phrases used (Minardi and Riley, 1997). Non-verbal communication, according to Ellis and Beattie (1986), contains the four elements of *prosodic*, paralinguistic, kinesics and standing features:

- Prosodic elements include intonation and rhythm. These can influence how the sender delivers the message and the receiver interprets it. For example, comprehension would alter if the sender of a message spoke quickly or slowly.
- Paralinguistic features include vocal but non-verbal expressions like 'mmm' or 'ahhh'. These can alter the way messages are communicated, particularly in relation to the prosodic features described above.
- Kinesic elements include body language, eye contact, posture or gestures. For example, different interpretations of messages would be transmitted by a sender who was trying to maintain eye contact as opposed to a sender who was looking at their feet.
- Standing features include factors such as appearance. Some people have preconceived notions of what practitioners who deliver health information should look like. This can include their dress, gender, ethnic group and other appearance-related factors.

Language and lexical content of the message is also important. Lexical content, which literally means the words, can be used positively or negatively. Using words from complex medical technology or abbreviating key terms can confuse messages and exclude the target audience, whereas repetition has been positively found to influence communication (Pechmann and Reibling, 2000).

As a health practitioner, the communication method will alter the importance of additional factors such as lexical content and body language. The communication process will dictate the aspects that are the most important. If you are sending every house in one area an information document about *prevention* of food-related illness and hence have minimal contact with the client group, your appearance and eye contact will be of little importance. If you are delivering a brief one-to-one intervention on stopping smoking in a health care setting your verbal communication, eye contact or appearance will be important.

COMMUNICATION IN HEALTH PROMOTION

Communication in health takes place on many constructs, including individual, group, community or mass media. Communication in health can be defined in much the same way as communication has generally been defined: a transactional process. Kreps (2003) summarises the addition of 'health' to the definition of the term communication as a 'resource' that allows health messages (e.g. prevention or awareness) to be used in the education and avoidance of ill health. This broad definition incorporates the fact that health communication can take place at many levels.

ACTIVITY 1.1
How are health promotion messages communicated?

There are a number of ways (or 'mediums') that can be used for communicating messages. Many of these can be used in communicating health messages.

1 Think of as many ways of communicating information as you can.
2 Which methods are most popularly used in communicating health promotion messages?

There are a range of communication channels that usually fall into four categories: interpersonal, organisational, community and public/mass. These are hierarchical in nature with interpersonal (one-to-one communication) reaching the least amount of people, and community reaching the whole population. Outside these channels are a variety of approaches which practitioners may use to achieve their goals. These include strategic communication, behaviour change communication, advocacy and social mobilisation. These methods are discussed in more detail in Chapter 2. Figure 1.3 illustrates these hierarchical channels. 'Interpersonal' communication is communication on a personal level. This includes one-to-one communication or small group communication. 'Organisational' communication includes communication in an organisation, both formal and informal. 'Community' communication includes media that are used in community settings, for example local radio and newspapers. 'Public/mass' communication is large-scale and includes national and international communication. Current research suggests that combining both interpersonal communication with communication at organisational or community level is more effective that mass media alone (see Chapter 4). Different health needs and priorities will require different styles of communication. For example, building negotiation skills for safer sex is more likely to be achieved through an interpersonal approach. Challenging incorrect beliefs about HIV transmission could be achieved

Type of channel	Definition of the channel	Examples of each channel
Interpersonal	Individual communication one-to-one	Health practitioner to patient/client, parent to child
Organisational	Locations where people live, work and play	Schools, workplaces, universities, supermarkets, places of worship or leisure centres
Community and public/mass	Wider media and wider community structures	Mass media channels, political or structural channels

Figure 1.3   Channels of communication examples

through a community approach. It has been noted however that this may not always be the case, for example those who are socially isolated and have limited social networks are less likely to use interpersonal communication and use mediated channels, i.e. television instead (Askelson et al., 2011), suggesting that hard-to-reach groups may be excluded from the more direct interpersonal communication channels.

MODELS AND THEORIES OVERVIEW

The UK government *Choosing Health: Making healthy choices easier* White Paper (DH, 2004) identifies one fundamental and important problem with health messages: that it is not a lack of information in health, but that it is 'inconsistent, uncoordinated and out of step' (DH, 2004: 21) with the way the population live their lives. This suggests perhaps that despite efforts from health practitioners, some messages are not as effective as they could be. Other authors argue that health practitioners can no longer provide knowledge, materials and support and assume the message will be sufficient for a behaviour change (Achterberg et al., 2010).

The Population Reference Bureau (2005) in the US suggests that human behaviour is the central factor in most leading causes of *mortality* and *morbidity*. They advocate that behaviour change strategies should be at the forefront of any attempts to reduce mortality and morbidity. Being able to predict behaviour makes it easier to plan an intervention (Naidoo and Wills, 2009). Therefore the first stage of any communication *campaign* is to analyse the behavioural aspects of the health problem (Atkin, 2001).

In addition it is proposed that if we can understand factors that influence behaviour 'we will be in a better position to devise strategies and formulate methods that will achieve our *health education* goals – no matter what our philosophy or what model we choose to follow' (Tones and Tilford, 1994: 83). *Theory* enables the practitioner to predict the outcomes of interventions and the relationships between internal and external variables. Underpinning communication in health promotion should be an understanding of how and why people change their behaviours and at what point of intervention it is best to target a message. This allows identification of the actions needed to change that behaviour and highlights the pathways of influence that hinder (or promote) that behaviour.

Theories do not specifically identify an intervention to follow. Instead they generate a series of ideas for a theory-led intervention to adopt. There are several theoretical models that identify influences in the behavioural change process. These can be selected according to what the practitioner wishes to achieve. The purpose of theory is to enable the successful exchange of information between the health promoter and the target audience (e.g. the individual, group, population). The success of this process is often down to the influence of a number of variables. These include, for example, the relationship between the communicator and audience (as described earlier), the message itself, how the message is sent and the audiences' beliefs, values, attitudes. Theory can therefore help predict and explain behaviours, assist in the targeting of information and predict the effect that information will have. It also allows practitioners to predict why the audience may not undertake a behaviour no matter how much assistance or encouragement is available.

Theory is often used to inform the groundwork for health promotion, but is usually given less attention (if any at all) during the implementation of programmes (Kobetz et al., 2005). For example, a study by Abraham et al. (2002) examined health promotion messages in safer sex promotion leaflets. They found that the majority of the leaflets examined did not include, or refer to, messages that targeted cognitions and actions that are most strongly related to condom use. This highlights a clear gap between the evidence-based research and practice in relation to designing safer sex promotion leaflets.

The application of theory to practice is not an easy step to make. Health promotion in the past has made use of theory sporadically, and often inconsistently. Jones and Donovan (2004) argue that practitioners frequently ignore theory, failing to use and implement theory-based interventions. They suggest that practitioners lack the skills and knowledge needed to operationalise the generic theories and models available. This is not to say that all health practitioners are ignorant of the importance and use of theory: some practitioners may have a clear theoretical knowledge but lack the time, resources, expertise or evidence base to implement their knowledge. In addition, guidance on theories is not always readily available, for example Achterberg et al. (2010) note that reviews on behaviour change often conclude interventions are effective without offering clarity on the intervention itself.

If communication is based on a theoretical model, some of the pitfalls associated with poor communication can be eliminated. Tones and Tilford (1994) argue that practitioners need a framework to make a clear selection of outcome indicators and to justify choice. In addition to this, it will provide a basis for best practice. In an age of cost-effectiveness alongside the move to evidence-based practice, the inclusion of theoretical models is a logical one. Kobetz et al. indicate that 'construction and strategic dissemination of finely tuned, theory-based health messages' (2005: 330) alongside making theory practically relevant is one of the keys to effective communication.

WHY USE THEORETICAL MODELS?

Models are derived from a simplified version of theory and can be used to guide the development of health promotion programmes. Theories and models are 'useful in planning, implementing and evaluating interventions' (Trifiletti et al., 2005: 299). Models in health promotion usually seek to include key elements important to behaviour and decision-making processes. In health promotion and health education, models are often borrowed from areas of social psychology or health communication and applied to health contexts.

Theories are valued in the field of health promotion because of their use in explaining influences on health alongside the ability to suggest ways where individual change could be achieved (Parker et al., 2004). They can be used to design and plan health promotion strategies and to generate decisions and solutions, ensuring that all variables are taken into consideration (Green and Tones, 2011). As Lewin surmises, 'there is nothing more practical than a good theory' (1951: 169).

PROBLEMS ASSOCIATED WITH A THEORY-BASED APPROACH

Although the evidence for using theory is difficult to refute, the use of theory is not without its problems. Green and Tones (2011) highlight the concern that theory objectifies human experience and through this process deviates from the main health promotion ethos of *holism* and *empowerment*. This means that a person is seen as someone who can be measured, analysed, adjusted or directed. This process opposes the idea of the person being seen as a whole, and is reductionist in nature. A broader concept of theory should perhaps be taken to alleviate the narrow, mechanistic focus that theory may have. Theory should be used as a means to guide the understanding of complex behaviour, rather than a rigid model that should be followed. Parker et al. (2004) suggest that designing interventions that attempt to focus on all aspects of a model may be both daunting and unrealistic. A suggestion is to focus on certain 'leverage points' or two or three stages in a model, for example 'subjective norms'. This may also be more practical for health campaigns.

The other key criticism of the theory-based approach is that structural, political and environmental factors are excluded in many theoretical models. Behaviour and influences on behaviour are altered by the wider societal context and theory often focuses on individuals only. This approach alone will not be effective without other enabling factors present to assist the facilitation of a behaviour change. It is important to remember when designing communication campaigns that supportive environments are available to facilitate change. Some evidence suggests that other approaches should be integrated alongside theoretical models such as social marketing and technology-based behaviour change models (Thompson and Ravia, 2011). Wider societal influences are sometimes difficult to control, for example government priorities, thus ambitions and objectives may need to be adjusted accordingly.

THEORIES

There are a multitude of theories that can be used in the communication of health. Four behaviour change theoretical models have been selected to cover a wide range of contexts for the purposes of this textbook. This is by no means a definitive coverage of the theoretical models available to the health practitioner. The models chosen have been selected for their suitability and popularity in the communication of health messages and their multiple uses from designing simple messages in leaflets to large-scale *mass media* campaigns. An additional theoretical model popularly used in campaigns is social marketing, which is explored in Chapter 4. The models selected encompass a variety of approaches that lend themselves to different communication projects in the health field.

In this chapter we will consider two types of theoretical models: cognitive theories and stage-step theories:

- *Cognitive theories* propose that a certain set of perceptions or beliefs will predict a behaviour. In the cognitive theories section the *theory of planned behaviour* (Ajzen, 1980) and *health belief model* (Becker, 1974) will be examined, and applied to the health communication context.
- *Stage-step theories* assume that the individual is not on a continuum (as they are in cognitive theories) but at a 'step' or 'stage'. Each step on the model is a move forward towards achieving the behaviour. Stage-step theories postulate that the individual goes through a process of change via a series of stages. Their format can be represented as cyclic or a literal series of steps. In this section the *transtheoretical model* or '*stages of change model*' (Prochaska and Diclemente, 1983), and the *process of behavioural change* (Population Communication Services/Center for Communication Programs, 2003) will be explored.

THEORY OF PLANNED BEHAVIOUR

This theory is the modified version of the *theory of reasoned action* (TRA) (Ajzen and Fishbein, 1980), where the additional variable of 'perceived behavioural control' has been added. The TRA originally proposed that any intervention attempting to change behaviour should focus on beliefs, as these influence *attitudes* and expectations and in turn influence intentions and behaviours. It was then proposed that behaviours are *not* under 'volitional control' and the model was re-visited and expanded to include 'perceived behaviour control' (Rutter and Quine, 2002). The TRA was revised to the *theory of planned behaviour* (TPB) (Ajzen, 1991). The TPB follows the same hypothesis as the TRA with the addition of 'behavioural control' as a determinant of behavioural intention and behavioural change (see Figure 1.4).

The TPB states that the closest determinant of behaviour is the intention to perform (or not perform) that behaviour (Jackson et al., 2005; Lavin and Groarke, 2005). The TPB's main determinant of behaviour is based on the person's intention to perform that behaviour, and intention is determined by three factors:

1 *Attitude to the behaviour:* the balancing of the pros/cons of performing the behaviour or the risks/rewards they associate with that choice.
2 *Subjective norm:* social pressure from significant others, for example peers, media or family.
3 *Perceived behavioural control:* the perception that person has about their ability to perform the behaviour.

This model can be represented more simplistically (see Figure 1.5). The simplistic version of the model proposes that the more positive the attitude, supportive the subjective norm and higher the perceived behavioural control *and* the stronger the intention, the more likely it is that a person will perform that behaviour (Lavin and Groarke, 2005).

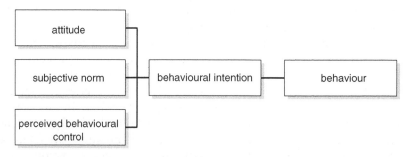

Figure 1.4   Theory of planned behaviour, adapted from Ajzen (1991)

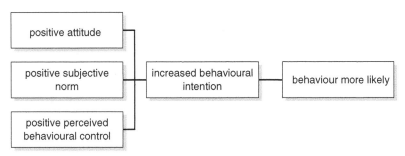

Figure 1.5 A simplistic view of the theory of planned behaviour hypothesis

ACTIVITY 1.3
The theory of planned behaviour in action

Daniel has been going to the gym for a few weeks as he wants to build up his muscles to make him look good. He has noticed no improvement so far in his muscles and the gym is costing him money. Daniel gets talking to one of the staff at the gym and explains how he feels and asks for some advice. The member of staff suggests he tries taking a supplement like steroids to help him build up his muscles. The staff member says he uses steroids and he feels great, and gained muscles in 'no time'.

1 Using the theory of planned behaviour, do you think Daniel will take the steroids?

The TPB has been widely applied in the context of understanding and predicting behaviour (Bledsoe, 2005). This includes using the determinants to predict behaviours such as fast-food consumption (Dunn et al., 2011) and parents as health promoters in obesity prevention (Andrews et al., 2010) alongside using the theory to design programme materials and interventions. For example Cottrell et al. (2010) use the TPB to develop culturally tailored materials for participation in a cardiovascular screening programme. Other examples use the theoretical framework to promote behaviour change in areas such as smoking cessation (Bledsoe, 2005), dental floss behaviour (Lavin and Groarke, 2005), promoting walking (Darker et al., 2010), increasing breakfast consumption (Kothe et al., 2011) and fruit and vegetable consumption (Kothe et al., 2012).

HEALTH BELIEF MODEL

Becker (1974) developed the *health belief model* (HBM) from the work of Rosenstock (1966). This model can be used as a pattern to evaluate or influence individual behavioural change. Figure 1.6 illustrates the health belief model.

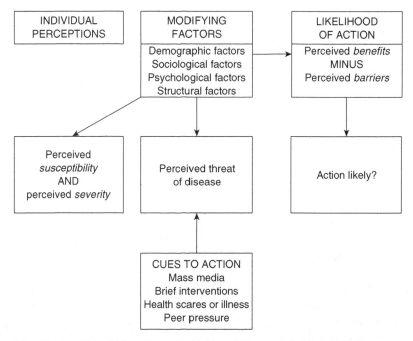

Figure 1.6 The health belief model, adapted from Rosenstock et al. (1988)

The model proposes that a person's behaviour can be predicted based on how vulnerable the individual considers themselves to be. 'Vulnerability' is expressed in the HBM through risk (perceived susceptibility) and the seriousness of consequences (severity). These two vulnerability variables need to be considered before a decision can take place. This means a person has to weigh up the costs/benefits or pros/cons of performing a behaviour. For example, this could include how 'susceptible' they feel they are to contracting an illness, for example mumps, and how 'severe' the consequences of having mumps is, or how 'susceptible' they are to an injury, for example falling off a bicycle without protective clothing, and how 'severe' the consequence will be. A person's decision to perform the health-promoting (or damaging) behaviour will be based on the outcome of this 'weighing up' process. More recently self-efficacy has been added to the health belief model which is the person's perceived confidence in their ability to perform a specific behaviour.

The HBM includes three 'weighing up' factors that need to take place for a behaviour change to occur:

1 *The person needs to have an 'incentive' to change their behaviour.* For example: an 'incentive' for a person to stop smoking could be the desire not to smoke around a new baby.

2 *The person must feel they are 'susceptible' to something, i.e. illness, if they do not perform the behaviour, and that the consequences of this will be 'severe'.* For example: by not taking preventive measures, such as compliance with anti-malarial drugs in a high malaria risk area, a person would feel that they would be putting themselves at 'risk' of contracting malaria.

3 *The person must believe change will have 'benefits', and these need to outweigh the 'barriers'.* For example: a person may believe that the benefits of using a bicycle helmet means they are less likely to have a serious head injury if they fall off their bicycle. They also identify the barriers to wearing one; they are cumbersome to carry throughout the day. In order for a change to be made the 'benefits' must outweigh the 'barriers'.

The HBM additionally suggests that there is a 'cue to action' to prompt the behaviour change process. This could be a conversation with a friend or a television programme. Alternatively, it could be an external prompt, such as moving employment. The prompt, however, has to be appropriate to that person.

The HBM also considers 'modifying factors' important to behaviour change. These include demographic variables, sociopsychological variables and structural variables that influence how a person perceives the disease severity, threats and susceptibility. Factors such as age, gender, peer pressure or prior contact with the disease also impact on the decision-making process.

The health belief model in action

Theo never wears a seatbelt. He has never crashed his car and thinks he is a good driver. He thinks seatbelts restrict his movement when driving and make him look 'uncool', and none of his friends wear seatbelts either.

Outcome: Using the HBM, the benefits Theo sees of wearing a seatbelt are minimal, and the barriers to wearing one are numerous (ruins his image, restricts movement, etc). It is likely that his decision will be that he does not wear a seatbelt as the costs (ruined image, restricted movement) outweigh the benefits (safety, injury prevention).

Case Study 1.1

This model, and elements from it – particularly 'perceived barriers' and 'perceived susceptibility' – has been used to predict a range of health behaviours. Moodi et al. (2011) for example use an education session which includes a lecture and film based on the HBM constructs to increase beliefs and perceived susceptibility to encourage breast screening examinations.

Other examples include the practice of adolescent health behaviours to prevent SARS (severe acute respiratory syndrome) (Wong and Tang, 2005), sexual behaviours and risk-taking (Lin et al., 2005), vaccination behaviour (De Wit et al., 2005), hypertension (Thackeray et al., 2011).

CRITICISMS OF COGNITIVE THEORIES

There are a number of criticisms of TPB and the HBM alongside other social cognitive models. Social cognitive models (the HBM in particular) emphasise a rational approach to behaviour and may exclude influential aspects such as friends, family or social norms. In addition an individual may not be a rational decision-maker who considers options before undertaking a behaviour; for example, Downing-Matibag and Geisinger (2009) note that in college students who 'hook up' (i.e. for the night) spontaneity undermines sexual efficacy. Careful consideration of which attitudes are more likely to lead to a behaviour intention may need additional thought as attitudes may not predict behaviours. The exclusion of the wider determinants of health from social cognitive models is a frequently cited criticism. Without identification of these wider determinants, some aspects of social cognitive models may not actually determine behaviour. In the TPB a focus on subjective norm ignores the other types of norms (i.e. individual perceptions of what is perceived as normal) (Paek et al., 2010).

Another criticism of these models is that they may be more suitable for small high-risk populations, rather than large-scale high-risk populations (Elder, 2001). Creating materials using theoretical constructs can be time and resource intensive, especially the collection of formative data needed to tailor constructs to materials (Cottrell et al., 2010).

The role of behavioural intentions may also be less important in non-Western cultures, as these theories assume a degree of autonomy alongside the Western biomedical model (King et al., 1995). In addition, the role of cultural contexts is missing and in non-Western populations these theories may be less culturally sensitive (Lin et al., 2005), especially if they promote individualism and remove emphasis on family or group behaviours (Airhihenbuwa and Obregon, 2000). Careful consideration of these aspects is needed before a model is chosen for use.

TRANSTHEORETICAL MODEL (OR 'STAGES OF CHANGE' MODEL)

The *transtheoretical model* (TTM), more frequently referred to as the 'stages of change' model, is a cyclic model developed by Prochaska and Diclemente (1983). The model suggests that people change their behaviour at certain stages in life, rather than making one major change. During these incremental stages, they consider whether or not to make changes to their behaviour (see Figure 1.7).

This cyclic model is based on the premise that people are at different levels of readiness to change and during the change process they move through a series of stages. People move from *precontemplation* (not ready to change) to

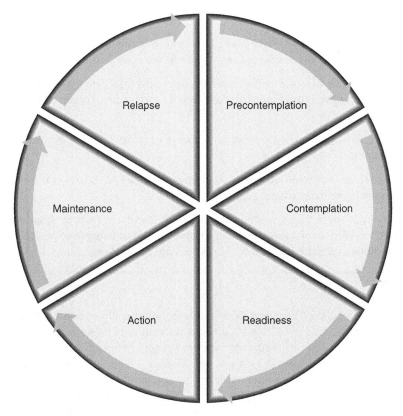

Figure 1.7   The transtheoretical model, adapted from Prochaska and Diclemente (1983)

contemplation (thinking of change), to *preparation* (getting ready to change), to *action* (performing the change), to *maintenance* (continuing the change), to *relapse* (abandoning changes and reverting to former behaviours). A person may start at any of these stages and may move between stages. Case Study 1.2 gives examples of these stages.

Physical activity and the transtheoretical model (TTM)

Precontemplation: A person who is sedentary and does not perceive any risks in being sedentary would be in the precontemplation phase of the TTM as they are not ready to change their behaviour. They cannot see any harm or risks in remaining sedentary.

(Continued)

Case Study 1.2

(Continued)

Contemplation: A person who is sedentary, but is aware of the risks of being sedentary and is perhaps considering the benefits or cons of exercise would be in the contemplation stage.

Preparation: Someone who is sedentary but has gone to the local gym to sign up for aerobics classes or is planning a walking route to work, would be in the preparation stage as they are getting ready to change.

Action: A person who has started exercising and has done so for a number of weeks would be in the action phase.

Maintenance: Once the person has been performing that behaviour (usually for six months or more), they are in the maintenance stage.

Relapse: At any of these stages, a person could 'fall off' this cycle. Perhaps despite planning they started to exercise for a few weeks before stopping. At this stage the person is seen to 'relapse' and then will move backwards to another stage of the cycle.

The TTM has been used extensively to guide behaviour change in a wide range of health promotion areas usually with a focus on simple behaviours. The model has frequently been used in targeting intervention programmes and *tailoring information* to appropriate stages of change. The model suggests that communication messages should be different for people in difference stages and even moving people from one stage to the next increases the likelihood of reaching the action stage (Paek et al., 2010). The model also offers opportunities for tailoring information using core concepts such as decisional balance (i.e. pros and cons), self-efficacy and processes of change (Haug et al., 2010). More recent research has suggested that if mediating variables allow groups to be collated together it is possible to collapse categories into three stages: precontemplation, contemplation/preparation and action/maintenance based on the differences in intention and behaviour (Di Noia and Prochaska, 2010; Lee et al., 2011). The rationale being that those who are in precontemplation are not intending to change behaviour, but those in contemplation/preparation are considering a change. Techniques are then targeted accordingly to the three groups. See Case Study 1.3 for an example of this.

It has also been said that it is a model that is 'simple, powerful, discerning and practical' (Brug et al., 2005). One of the most appealing aspects of the TTM to practitioners is its simplicity. Although originally designed for smoking interventions, recently the TTM has been used in areas that include promoting fruit and vegetable consumption (Ruud et al., 2005), emergency preparedness (Paek et al., 2010), contraceptive use (Lee et al., 2011), dietary change (Di Noia and Prochaska, 2010; Di Noia et al., 2008; Salehi et al., 2011) and physical activity in older people (Kirk et al., 2010).

The transtheoretical model (TTM) in action

Case Study 1.3

A dietary intervention programme to increase fruit and vegetable uptake divided the stages of change into three groups.

Precontemplation: Consciousness raising, dramatic relief, environmental re-evaluation processes for enhancing awareness of intake levels, promoting acceptance for need to change.

Contemplation/preparation: Self re-evaluation and self-liberation strategies to increase confidence in the ability to increase fruit and vegetable intake, resolve ambivalence regarding commitment to act, facilitate specific plans to achieve outcomes.

Action/maintenance: Reinforcement management, counter-conditioning, stimulus control processes for promoting problem solving in situations that challenge efforts to maintain intake.

(Di Noia and Prochaska, 2010; Di Noia et al., 2008)

PROCESS OF BEHAVIOUR CHANGE (PoBC)

An alternative model to the TTM is the *process of behaviour change* (PoBC) model. Described by the Population Communication Services/Center for Communication Programs (2003) in the US, this model recognises communication as a process where people can move between the stages of the PoBC framework. Different messages are sought depending on where the person is on the PoBC framework. The main difference between the PoBC and the TTM is that the model is not seen as circular, but as a series of 'steps' where a person moves upwards towards a final goal. In the PoBC people move through the following steps (and see Figure 1.8):

- Preknowledge: When a person is unaware of any risks or problems associated with their behaviour.
- Knowledgeable: When a person is aware of the problem and of the risks attached to their behaviour.
- Approving: When a person is in favour of changing their behaviour.
- Intending: When a person is intending to take action to change their behaviour.
- Practising: When the intended behaviour is being practised.
- Advocating: When the new behaviour is being implemented and when a person then advocates that behaviour to another.

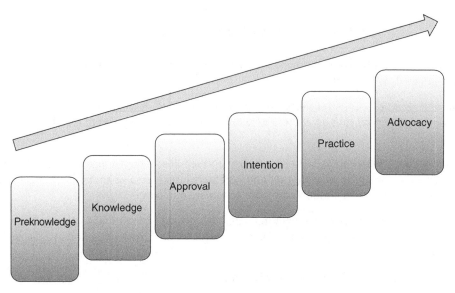

Figure 1.8   The process of behaviour change (PoBC) model, based on Population
Communication Services/Center for Communication Programs

ACTIVITY 1.4
The process of behaviour change (PoBC) model in action

You are working in a local community and you want to raise awareness about new
recycling bins that are now available for community use. You are trying to encourage
those that use the recycling bins already to advocate using them to others.

1   What would people need to do at each step on the PoBC model to achieve this?

CRITICISMS OF STAGE-STEP THEORIES

Stage-step models have been criticised for a number of reasons. Practitioners and the
targeted individual's idea of which stage the person is in may conflict or be inaccurate (Brug
et al., 2005). Some people may place themselves at wrong stages on the model, or their
actions are interpreted as being in a different phase than they actually are. A review also
found that the TTM is used inconsistently in the development of programme design
(Hutchison et al., 2009). This may lead to limited success. West (2005) argues that some of
the stages are 'soft' options, for example moving from precontemplation to contemplation

is not a strong move to change behaviour as there is no measurable behaviour change. West (2005) also argues that the TTM assumes that the individual has made a rational plan (e.g. to quit smoking) that does not take into account entrenched habits or irrationality. Aspects included in social cognitive models, for example *self-efficacy*, attitudes or subjective norms, are not included in the TTM.

Brug et al. (2005) debate a variety of aspects of the TTM. They consider that it is difficult to apply to complex behaviour, especially if environmental variables are also needed to change (e.g. behaviours that need money or transportation). They also argue that the TTM is more likely to change short-term behaviours than long-term. Effectiveness of this model is also varied as a stand-alone theory (Callaghan et al., 2010) and campaigns may need to utilise a range of other theories and strategies alongside the TTM for success.

PRACTICAL IMPLICATIONS: WHICH THEORETICAL MODEL?

There are many models and theories in use in the respective disciplines of communication and health promotion. Some of these are of more use to the health practitioner than to others. It is not simply the case that 'one model fits all'. Communication in the health setting uses different methods, with different messages for different audiences. All the models described (alongside some not described – see the additional reading section at the end of this chapter) have the potential to be utilised effectively in the communication of health promotion campaigns.

There are no set guidelines for practitioners to help them select which model to use. It is possible that a 'theory of the problem approach' may be useful, which involves identifying the health issues and then locating the main theories that could be useful and selecting the most appropriate one for understanding the causal factors and processes of specific health behaviours (Mier et al., 2010).

Green and Tones (2011) list a series of questions that the practitioner could consider before selecting models:

- Does it include all relevant variables?
- Does it make logical sense to use this model in this particular situation?
- Has it been used elsewhere for a similar purpose?
- Are there any studies to illustrate its use in the chosen area?

Difficulties may also stem from an overlap between models, for example Paek et al. (2010) suggest focusing on individual perceptions, self-efficacy, subjective norm and increasing the stage of preparation may all be effective approaches for improving public emergency preparedness. Berndt et al. (2011) note that perceived barriers, perceived benefits, levels of concern (susceptibility), personal and group norms contribute to sun screen use. Both of these examples highlight that variables span more than one behaviour change model. It is possible therefore that more than one model is selected for inclusion in an intervention. Selection of theoretical models can also be based on personal choice, target group, funding, time, influences of stakeholders, size of project and behaviours that are being targeted. Figure 1.9 illustrates each theoretical model with the common client/person contact that it has been used for. The figure also shows settings where this model has been applied and the appropriate topic interventions. This is by no means an exhaustive list of every setting or topic these models have been used for, and practitioners should investigate their own topic fully before selecting a model(s) of choice to use in their communication project.

Model	Key variables	Example settings	Examples of topic interventions
Theory of planned behaviour (TPB)	Attitude Subjective norm Perceived behavioural control Behavioural intentions Behaviour	Group settings: church, schools, universities, workplaces Wider settings: communities, towns	• Physical activity • Accident/injury prevention • Tobacco uptake • Oral health • Alcohol/drug misuse
Health belief model (HBM)	Perceived susceptibility Perceived severity Perceived threat Perceived benefits Perceived barriers Cue to action	Group settings: church, schools, universities, workplaces	• Preventive behaviour: • Physical activity • Sexual healtη • Vaccinations • Dietary changes
Transtheoretical model (TTM) or process of behaviour change (PoBC)	Precontemplation/ preknowledge Contemplation/knowledge Readiness/approval/ intention Action/practice Maintenance Advocacy Relapse	Medical settings: general practice, dentists, pharmacies Group settings: schools, universities, workplaces Service settings: stop smoking groups, screening	• Tobacco • Physical activity • Alcohol/drug misuse • Accident/injury prevention • Cancer screening • Nutrition/diet

Figure 1.9   Examples of theoretical models that can be used in practice by group, setting and intervention

PRACTICAL IMPLICATIONS: GETTING STARTED

Often models assume some pre-contact with the client/person before an intervention can take place. For example, if you can identify the barriers that the client groups experience or the attitudes that are shared in relation to behaviours, it is easier to identify the topics to address. Communicating with your chosen target group before your intervention commences enables you to foster a more *bottom-up approach* to health communication, facilitating a transactional information exchange process. Data can be collected using a range of methods such as rapid appraisal techniques, focus groups, questionnaires and so on.

If you cannot access the target group beforehand, this makes things more complex. How do you know that your intervention will be successful if you cannot ask any questions before you get started? Also, the planned intervention will be taking a *top-down approach*, communication will be one-sided and may exclude the very group you are trying to reach. The principles of evidence-based practice (see Chapter 7) alongside researching other campaigns in your chosen area, will be of help here.

THE THEORY OF PLANNED BEHAVIOUR IN PRACTICE

Application of the TPB is particularly useful when there is access to a group first, allowing the mapping of major beliefs that may help or hinder performance of behaviours. One of the other advantages of this model is the inclusion of the 'subjective norm' allowing focus on peer or family influences. Other studies suggest that variables such as perceived behavioural control might be appropriate, for example in driving behaviours (Elliott and Armitage, 2009) and smoking intentions (Murnaghan et al., 2010). Case Study 1.4 illustrates the theory of planned behaviour in the context of speeding.

Theory of planned behaviour in action

Below is one example of campaign materials that aim to target subjective norms.
Elliott and Armitage (2009) targeted speeding in drivers. Their materials had this message:
Do the people important to you really want you or themselves to be involved in an accident? Many drivers say that a reason why they sometimes drive faster than the speed limit is because they think other people would want them to do so. Drivers may think that people important to them, or people whose views they respect, would approve of them driving faster than the speed limit. However, is this really the case? It is a fact that increases in driving speed will increase the risk of a road traffic accident. It is also a fact that increases in driving speed will increase the severity of an accident, were it to occur.

Case Study 1.4

THE HEALTH BELIEF MODEL IN PRACTICE

The HBM can be applied to a variety of health behaviours. Interventions using this model usually aim to influence the 'perceived threat of disease' variable and hence change the susceptibility/severity balance. The main way of doing this tends to be directing information that has an emotional appeal or contains a strong fear or emotional response. Topics such as drink-driving, accidents, domestic violence, substance misuse (particularly illegal drugs) and road safety are good examples of this and often lend themselves to creating an emotional response to the topic (see Chapter 4 for more on this).

As the HBM suggests, barriers may be more important than benefits (Janz and Becker, 1984; Lajunen and Räsänen, 2004), barriers may also provide a focus for targeting communication. For example, studies indicate that concern about pain in *screening* for preventive behaviours (Byrd et al., 2004; Weinberg et al., 2004, in colon and cervical screening) can be a significant barrier to overcome. If a practitioner can identify barriers to performing behaviours, an intervention can focus on these to promote a behaviour change.

Other aspects of the HBM have also been found to be associated with behaviours. Moser et al. (2005) found perceived benefits to be a predictor of fruit and vegetable consumption. Lin et al. (2005) suggest that self-efficacy is a strong predictor of sexual behaviour, whereas Weitkunat et al. (2003) found 'perceived threat' to be an important aspect of dietary behaviour. De Wit et al. (2005) promote the use of perceived susceptibility and severity as being important components of interventions, thus illustrating that parts of the TPB could be used in practice. See Case Study 1.5 for an example of perceived severity/susceptibility in action.

Case Study 1.5

The health belief model in practice – asthma

A Community Action Against Asthma (CAAA) example (Parker et al., 2004).

As part of the CAAA, the HBM was used to target information to children with asthma and their care-givers, given by a community environmental specialist (CES). Education messages were aimed at increasing perceived susceptibility and increasing the care-givers' perceived severity by identifying with the care-givers different types of environmental allergens or irritants and how they can affect children's asthma. To increase care-givers' perceived benefits, the CES practitioner explained links between reducing environmental allergens or irritants and ways to do this (cleaning, etc.) and the benefit to the child. In response to perceived barriers, provision of vacuum cleaners, cleaning supplies, mattress covers, etc. were made available alongside referral to appropriate agencies to help with issues such as childcare.

APPLICATION OF THE TRANSTHEORETICAL MODEL TO PRACTICE

Application of the TTM (or the PoBC) is particularly useful when there is access to the client group first allowing the mapping of individuals to stages, preferably through face-to-face involvement. For example, the TTM provides an opportunity for stage-tailored information, such as tailoring newsletters (Ruud et al., 2005) or brief advice. First, questions will need to be asked of the client. These should include questions about past behaviour, current behaviour and future intentions, including current knowledge and practice. The questions can be brief and allow the practitioner to apply a stage to a person's response. Once the stage on the TTM has been decided, the level of action will then be appropriate to that stage. This may consist of doing very little (not everyone is going to want to change). As behaviour changes, there may be a need to assess 'stages' at each encounter with the person.

The types of action you may take could include:

- Precontemplation: providing information, highlighting benefits.
- Contemplation: examining ways of overcoming barriers, including access, cost, transport, time or fear.
- Preparation: support for any last-minute problems, providing additional advice.
- Action/maintenance: continue to support positive choice made.
- Relapse: advice to try again when a person is ready, alongside re-checking the stage a person is at.

Case Study 1.6 illustrates an example of the TTM in practice, and how these stages can be used in campaign design.

The stages of change in action – sexual health education and condom use for postpartum women

Lee et al. (2011) utilised the TTM by splitting the cycle into three phases. Women were stage matched and divided into three groups: precontemplation, contemplation and preparation/action. All groups received a self-help booklet.

In the precontemplation phase they received techniques including dramatic consciousness and decisional balance (pros and cons) and were encouraged to ask questions.

In the contemplation stage they received motivational interviews, self-efficacy strategies, decisional balance and self re-evaluation. In the preparation/action stage the focus was on self-liberation, and evaluating and strengthening techniques to promote contraceptive health.

Case Study 1.6

ACTIVITY 1.5
How are health promotion messages communicated?

In adolescent 'hook ups' (i.e. casual one night relationships) there is evidence that students' sexually efficacious behaviour could be promoted by programmes that involve role-playing videos or activities that teach them how to effectively negotiate the use of protection (Downing-Matibag and Geisinger, 2009).

Based on the behaviour change models described in this chapter:

1 Which variables would you target in a behaviour change model to promote safer sexual relationships?
2 What sort of messages would you target at the constructs of this model to promote safer sexual relationships?

CONCLUSION

Health promotion campaigns should be planned and designed utilising models that can best predict possible outcomes of behaviours based on the available evidence of effectiveness. This will ensure that appropriate and influential social cognitive constructs are targeted that best predict behaviours. This chapter has drawn attention to a variety of theoretical models that can be used in full or part to help inform health communication programmes, although there are others that are equally important in health promotion, and that practitioners may prefer to use.

Although theoretical models do not provide a full explanation of every factor in the behaviour change process, they identify potential factors or leverage points that may influence decisions that can help in the targeting and structuring of communication. Current thinking suggests that theory-based approaches may not achieve large effects if they are used alone, but make up the bigger picture of health communication strategies and should be used alongside other communication techniques such as social marketing or advocacy techniques.

Summary

- This chapter has discussed the role and application of theoretical models in health promotion practice.
- Two cognitive models, the theory of planned behaviour and the health belief model, and two stage-step models, the transtheoretical model and perceived behavioural control model, were described and applied to practice.
- The advantages of using theory were highlighted alongside criticisms of the theoretical approach.
- The use of theory in practice was examined alongside the application of theoretical models to health promotion practice.

ADDITIONAL READING

Theoretical models are discussed in more detail by a variety of authors.

A lengthy chapter on theory and practice is available in Green J and Tones K (2011) *Health Promotion: Planning and strategies*, 2nd edition. Sage, London.

A good introduction to all key health promotion theories is Nutbeam D, Harris E and Wise M (2010) *Health Promotion Theory in a Nutshell*. McGraw Hill, Maidenhead.

A good guide for practitioners working in hands-on healthy behaviour areas with theoretical links is Upton D and Thirlaway K (2010) *Promoting Healthy Behaviour*. Pearson, London.

2

SOCIAL AND PSYCHOLOGICAL FACTORS

NOVA CORCORAN AND SUE CORCORAN

Learning objectives:

- Examine social and psychological factors that influence health promotion and health communication in a health context.
- Explore ways social and psychological factors can impact on health promotion and the implications of this for communication in health promotion.
- Identify methods of communicating with different audiences taking into consideration their social and psychological characteristics and utilising the example of attitudinal change.

Chapter 1 described communication in health as a multi-level transactional process of information exchange in a health-related context. In order for this transactional process to be effective, a number of key factors need to be taken into account when starting the design of a health communication campaign. This chapter will consider 'social' and 'psychological' factors of the target group for effective communication planning. Social factors include variables such as age, gender, ethnicity, religion and education. Psychological factors refer to attitudes, beliefs and values. This chapter will examine each in turn and consider how these factors influence communication and the campaign process. It will also investigate the ways these factors impact on effective communication in health, and consider ways to utilise these differences when targeting health promotion interventions. Particular attention will be focused on how the target group characteristics can impact on campaigns, alongside how to influence attitudes and behaviours focusing on these factors.

THE TARGET GROUP

According to Morrell, 'communication is linked to the social environment in which it is taking place' (2001: 33). From this premise Morrell identifies a variety of social factors which can effect communication, including age, gender, social class, ethnicity, social status, language, power and social relations (such as roles or scripts). Thus, in the wider environment that communication takes place, there are influential factors which impact on the communication process. These are all factors, or traits, that each person has, and will vary between person to person. These factors will influence a variety of processes in communication, including how, when and where communication is received and how it will be acted upon. Figure 2.1 illustrates how some of these factors influence a person. In the inner circle are social factors such as age, gender or ethnic group. In the middle circle are psychological factors such as attitudes, *values* or beliefs, and the outer circle contains the wider environment incorporating factors that impact on both social and psychological factors.

As Figure 2.1 suggests, social factors impact on psychological factors and the attitudes, beliefs and values that each person has. This suggests, in the planning stages of health promotion, that these factors will need to be taken into account. For example, social factors can influence how individuals perform protective behaviours, such as regular physical activity. Different groups will perform this behaviour in different ways; young age groups might partake in all physical activity in a school setting, older age groups might use the gym. Social factors also impact on an individual's attitudes, beliefs or values to performing behaviours and thereby need high priority in any proposed health communication project.

ACTIVITY 2.1
Differences in health behaviours

A 17-year-old male from a lower socioeconomic class will probably not perform the same health-related behaviours as a 17-year-old female from a higher socioeconomic class. For example, in relation to driving, males are more likely to drug-drive and drink-drive than their female counterparts (Neale et al., 2001) and are also more likely to have an accident on the road (Lancaster and Ward, 2002).

1 What different health behaviours might there be between a 25-year-old Asian female and a Black African 60-year-old female?
2 What different health behaviours might there be between a 50-year-old male of no religious affiliation and a 50-year-old female from a Muslim faith?

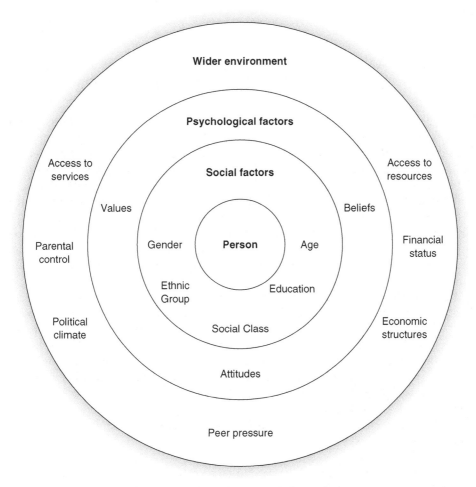

Figure 2.1 Social and psychological factors and the wider environment

The assumption, based on differences in social factors, is that the more pre-planning that takes these factors into consideration, the more realistic the outcomes of the intervention will be, and the more likely that the target group will be responsive to an intervention.

Although groups can share similar characteristics (e.g. age or ethnic group), psychological factors are frequently pertinent to an individual and often internalised so they cannot be seen by others (thus making our 17-year-old in Activity 2.1 different from other 17-year-olds). Psychological factors include attitudes, beliefs and values and can influence a person's communication and likelihood of adherence or reception to that communication internally. Some groups can share similar attitudes, beliefs or values, but if a mix of social factors is also added, it becomes less likely that all the people in that group will be identical.

THE RELEVANCE OF SOCIAL AND PSYCHOLOGICAL FACTORS TO COMMUNICATION

Populations can differ in terms of their trust, use and preference of information sources in health communication sources. Health media use is patterned by ethnicity, language and social class (Viswanath and Ackerson, 2011) as well as other social factors such as age and sex. Differences are complex, for example demographic differences have been identified in protective behaviours during a pandemic. Being female, older, more educated and non-white are associated with a higher chance of adopting protective behaviours (Bish and Michie, 2010). This suggests a complexity to social factors that influence behaviour. This is supported by Sharangpani et al. (2011) who also suggest demographic characteristics are an important influence in protective behaviours for pandemic influenza.

Although this textbook will look at each factor in turn, in practice psychological and social factors combine together (as shown in Figure 2.1). Hopman-Rock et al. (2004) provide an examination of determinants of participation in a health exercise and education programme transmitted via television in the Netherlands. They found that higher age (older), female gender, positive intention, knowledge and lower barriers were associated with participation in the health education programme. This example illustrates that links between social and psychological factors need careful consideration. There are two main ways social and psychological factors should be identified when planning and targeting health communication interventions:

1   Social and psychological factors need to be taken into consideration when targeting health promotion interventions. Questions to ask include:

   • Which groups perform (or do not perform) certain behaviours?
   • What are the needs of the target group?
   • What benefits might the target group experience if they perform a behaviour?
   • What barriers do the target group experience to performing a behaviour?

2 Social and psychological factors need to be taken into consideration when planning which communication methods to use. Questions to ask include:

- Which medium will appeal to this group?
- What messages need to be transmitted to this group?
- How will messages be framed to appeal to this group?

The more attention that goes into mapping these variables, the more likely the health communication will be relevant, appropriate and well targeted. This strategy is in line with recommendations made by the former *Health Development Agency* (HDA) (2005) in the UK, which suggests targeted and tailored information is imperative for an effective and successful health promotion intervention.

SOCIAL FACTORS OVERVIEW

This section considers age, sex and gender, socioeconomic class and education levels, ethnicity and culture.

Age

The age of the target group influences information preferences for health promotion messages. Factors such as the language or dialect that is used in a health promotion intervention can have an effect on the target group. Different age groups use, understand and interpret language differently.

Different age groups seek health information from different sources. Research shows that television is cited by younger age groups as a health information preference and there were decreasing reports of the use of television as a source of health information with age (Kakai et al., 2003). Kakai et al. also found that newspapers and magazines were perceived as an important source of information in younger age groups, and health professionals were seen as a valuable source of information in older age groups and this importance increased with age. Peterson et al. (2005) found in a physical activity campaign that television was effective in reaching 18- to 30-year-olds, although it had less impact on intention to exercise than in those who saw the advertisements on billboards and *bus wraps*. This suggests careful analysis of information preferences that are most likely to lead to action is valuable.

A study by Graff et al. (2004) found differences in attitudes to the Internet with lower age groups (17–19) reporting more positive attitudes than older age groups (21–32). Again, this highlights the need to consider the target group in detail, rather than making estimations that everyone in the 'young adult' age range behaves identically. Age can also correlate with knowledge and Marek et al. (2011) note that older age (and being female) correlate with better knowledge of sexually transmitted infections (STIs).

Age can influence reactions to message content. For example, Henley and Donovan (2003) illustrate that scare tactics in the media have little effect on older females, who respond significantly more to non-threats, whereas older males were seen to respond more to scare tactics. Other research suggests age-related complexities. For example in a drug use campaign different age groups reported different drug use levels with campaign awareness (Scheier and Grenard, 2010). The wording of health promotion messages will also need consideration. How a health product is labelled or packaged has an impact on different audiences. Latimer et al. (2012) note that adolescent smokers find generic warning labels on cigarette packets uninteresting and irrelevant, and only pay attention or think about these labels some of the time suggesting other preventive strategies may need to be considered for younger smokers.

Sex and gender

Sex and gender are important components of the communication process. Sex differences determine the medium and message sought for health communication. Gender, although often the term used to classify men and women, is actually not the biological difference between men and women (sex) but the masculine or feminine *qualities* that a male or female may possess. A study by Kakai et al. (2003) found that females are more likely to obtain their health information from health care professionals and males from newspapers, suggesting a difference in information-seeking preferences. Peterson et al. (2005) postulate that in promoting physical activity to women in the 18–30 age range, television was an effective way of reaching this group. Bessinger et al. (2004) consider multi-media exposure on knowledge and use of condoms in Uganda, and indicate exposure to general media messages regarding STIs were more likely to predict a female likelihood of using a condom at the last sexual encounter but not male. Although they additionally propose that men were more responsive to a radio message than women. Walsh et al. (2011) suggest that nutritional advice sort by male schoolboy rugby players was mostly sought from coaches or magazines. Other studies suggest that men receive health information through lay media, friends or family members (Ferrante et al., 2011). This highlights complex differences between channel and content of the message in relation to audience preference and exposure.

Marston (2004) suggests that there are differences between the way men and women communicate and want to be communicated with and that these are often socially determined. Investigation into what is best for the target group needs consideration, and if the target group is mixed, messages and mediums will need to be acceptable and effective with both groups. For example, it will be difficult to foster communication between sexes if topics being covered are traditionally taboo. Sivaram et al. (2005) found in India that spousal communication around the topic of sex and sexual health was minimal, although unmarried men were more likely to discuss sex and sexual health. It might be more appropriate in the first instance to develop interventions that focus on unmarried men's discourse in sexual health, rather than promoting mixed-sex discourse that is more challenging. Akhund and Yousafzai (2011) found that women's groups have proved to be a workable option for the delivery of health care interventions in some developing countries. This may be partly due to the acceptability and accessibility of the location, for example a safe and open setting for discussion around health issues.

Socioeconomic class and education levels

Language, medium and location of where an audience accesses health messages can vary depending on social structure or class and education levels. Different social classes use language in different ways, and education levels can be influential in how people respond to health communication. Problematically social determinants like socioeconomic status may increase communication inequalities, as socioeconomic status can influence health seeking behaviours. Those with higher education levels tend to seek more information than lower social classes, and where information that is located suggests differences in channels and format preferences (Galarce et al., 2011).

Little educational background may mean difficulties in learning new facts or remembering knowledge (Povlsen et al., 2005). Low education levels may also mean only partial understanding of complex messages. Niederdeppe et al. (2011) found that smokers with low levels of education and income less often recall advertisements focused on how to quit, and perceive them less effective than ads using graphic imagery or personal testimonials to convey why they quit. This suggests a preference both in the educational message itself, and the imagery used depending on social class. Social class may also impact on appeal of messages. Spotswood and Tapp (2010) suggest that those from a working-class background differ in their inactivity levels due to class-related differences. These were centred around having fewer social bonds, that physical activity was not a norm in working-class life and lower levels of perceived efficacy. The authors suggest that messages such as exercise is good for you or is fun are unlikely to have an impact based on how exercise is perceived by this group.

Preference of information source has also been found to be influenced by education levels and it has been suggested that lower education may be associated with not being able to access health information easily, for example lack of access to the Internet may impact on health information. Chivu and Reidpath (2010) note that the relationship between area deprivation and the impact of health promotion (i.e. having a lesser impact) may be linked to access of health promotion information. They note that the odds of requesting health promotion materials in schools are less in the most deprived areas. Not requesting information is associated with lack of exposure to health messages. This is supported by Taylor-Clark et al. (2010), who note that in Hurricane Katrina lower social classes were less exposed to emergency information and orders and they suggest fewer social networks are a partial cause.

ACTIVITY 2.2
Messages for education levels

Have a look at these two websites around diabetes. Diabetes UK at www.diabetes.org.
uk and NHS diabetes available at www.diabetes.nhs.uk.

1   Which do you think is easier to navigate for someone in a lower social class?
2   Which do you think is more appealing to lower or higher education levels? Why?

Ethnicity and culture (see also Chapter 3)

Ethnicity and culture are complex terms and although these concepts are explored
in depth in Chapter 3 it is helpful to define them here. Ethnicity is a term used to
categorise groups based on cultural characteristics such as shared ancestry, religion
or language. Race is a term used to distinguish biologically between groups. Culture
can reflect both of these concepts and is a 'system of shared understanding that
shapes and, in turn, is shaped by experience' (Caprio et al., 2008: 2214).

It has been acknowledged that individual needs of minority ethnic groups are
not always met adequately in the health promotion context. Problems linked
with *stereotyping* behaviours and beliefs may be prevalent and recognition of
traditional practices and beliefs may be important to communicating with some
groups. Different cultural beliefs can also mean that traditional Western forms of
communicating health information are inadequately designed (Povlsen et al., 2005)
and therefore do not have the desired impact on the target group. Language barriers
in particular are important in health promotion work. They can contribute to poor
health communication and present a disparity between those who can speak the
predominant language and those who cannot.

Identification of characteristics that distinguish ethnic groups is difficult as culture,
religion, age and gender also interact on individuals and communities thereby creating
no single homogeneous group. There is some evidence to suggest differences in
information preference and perceptions of health although this information is sparse.
For example Sugerman et al. (2011) suggest in an obesity prevention opinion poll that
Latinos reported receiving the most information from television, and Hmong from
the radio. A different study found that Spanish-speaking Hispanics were more likely
that non-Hispanic whites to pay attention to and trust health messages from the radio.
Non-Hispanic blacks were more likely than non-Hispanic whites to pay attention
to and trust messages on the television (Viswanath and Ackerson, 2011). A study in
Malaysia examining public sources of information for pandemic influenza notes ethnic
differences in information sources with Malays preferring television and Chinese and
Indians preferring newspapers and health care providers (Wong and Sam, 2010). Other
studies highlight the complexities in relation to ethnicities and behaviours, for example
Griffith et al. (2011) highlight the complexities in ethnicity in relation to attitudes and

experiences in sex such as information sources, contraception use and discussions of sex which varied between ethnicity and gender. These examples serve to illustrate the complexities of information preferences and health communication needs to be dedicated to meeting the differing requirements of different ethnic groups. Culture is explored in more depth in Chapter 3.

SOCIAL FACTORS AND HEALTH PROMOTION PRACTICE

Communication should be designed to take into consideration the range of social factors of the target group. In practice social factors come as a package. For example Oyediran et al. (2011) found that level of education, place of residence in childhood, region, religious affiliation, economic status index and exposure to mass media were associated with sexual experience and use of protective measures, i.e. condom use. Large-scale mass media campaigns are designed to take into account the social factors of the audience and will have clear age, gender, socioeconomic status/ education levels and ethnic groups in mind in the design of a campaign. Wanyoni et al. (2011) in a review of face-to-face tailored messages in patient settings suggest that health practitioners should take time to discover patients' psychosocial characteristics to provide tailored health messages. This would suggest researching the influence of these social variables on health outcomes.

ACTIVITY 2.3
Who is the message designed for?

Look at Figure 2.2 'Clear on cancer' which is designed to raise awareness and facilitate conversation with GPs on bowel cancer. Consider the image being used (i.e. Dr Rajive Mitra) and the main message of the poster. Consider who the poster is designed for under the following headings:

1 What age is the poster aimed at?
2 What sex is the poster aimed at?
3 What socioeconomic status is the material aimed at?
4 What education level is the material aimed at?
5 What ethnicity is the material aimed at?

Once you have completed this task look at Figure 4.2 in Chapter 4 and ask the questions above in reference to this poster.

6 What are the similarities and differences in design between the two posters in terms of the target group?

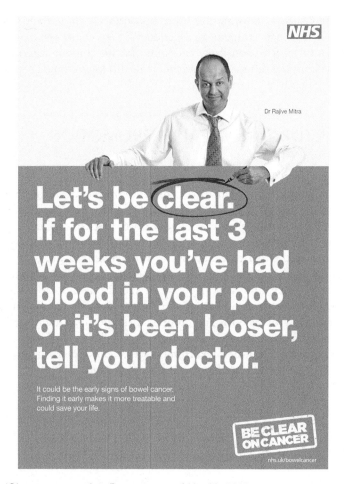

Figure 2.2 'Clear on cancer', © Department of Health 2012

It is possible to target more than one group at any one time with the same campaign design as small, segmented population groups may not be a particularly cost effective focus of a campaign. Just targeting one group may exclude other important groups. An example could be a target group of older male and female adults that have differing information needs and preferences for cancer screening information. Although the main campaign strategy might be similar, for example encouraging uptake of screening for cancer(s) targeting those who have never been screened, the campaign could be tailored to more specific target groups. For example using community resources could include the locations where groups frequent (coffee shops, churches, social clubs, etc.) and information preferences, i.e. radio in females or newspapers in males, can be accommodated to best fit with target group needs.

Netto et al. (2010) notes five principles for adapting behavioural interventions in ethnic minority communities which can be adapted and used to assist in tailoring campaign strategies for more than one target group:

- Use community resources to publicise the intervention and increase accessibility.
- Identify and address barriers to participation.
- Develop communication strategies that are sensitive to language use and information requirements.
- Work with values (i.e. cultural, religious, family) that promote or hinder behaviour change.
- Accommodate varying degrees of cultural identification or group identity, i.e. social or group norms.

PSYCHOLOGICAL FACTORS OVERVIEW

Previously, discussion has focused on social factors, which are externally visible factors. Psychological factors are internal variables which influence a person's decision to perform an action or behaviour. In the case of health these psychological variables are linked to the performance of health promotion or health preventive actions and behaviours. In health promotion the three factors that have received the most attention are attitudes, beliefs and values. An understanding of these factors can assist in the formulation of effective interventions in health promotion. Attitudes have received the most attention and are arguably the most influential of the three factors, thus many health promotion campaigns have aimed to change, influence or challenge attitudes. A number of campaigns based in theoretical models have also sought to examine attitudes, beliefs and values and their role in behaviour change.

Attitudes, beliefs and values can be hard to observe, although a person's beliefs and values often predict an attitude, and this can then be observed by others in the form of behaviour (Morrell, 2001). Thus we should be able to observe behaviour and formulate what the attitudes, beliefs and values might be, bearing in mind that psychological factors do not always predict a behavioural outcome and can be unpredictable in nature. In addition the complexities of a variety of social cognitive variables may be equally important (see Chapter 1). Baron-Epel (2010) found in a study examining attitudes and beliefs to breast cancer in a multi-ethnic population that subjective norm, fatalism, fear of breast cancer and perceived effectiveness of mammography were highlighted by different groups, which are all factors that have a complex relationship to and with attitudes, beliefs and values.

ACTIVITY 2.4
Psychological variables and MMR

The MMR vaccine remains a controversial vaccine despite a wide range of scientific research to refute claims of links to autism and other health-related issues.

What is your attitude towards the MMR vaccine? What do you believe about the health problems linked to the vaccine? If you have children would you vaccinate them? What information are you basing your decisions on?

ATTITUDES

Attitude change is often considered to be an important part of health promotion in the move to encouraging individuals to adopt healthy practices. Attitudes occupy a central role in health promotion practice as they are closely linked to beliefs and values. What attitudes are and how they can be changed or influenced has always retained a lively debate and some suggest that the attitudinal approach in health promotion campaigns is underutilised (Panagopoulou et al., 2011).

Attitudes have been defined as relatively stable with consistent outcomes and research suggests that the relationship between attitude and behaviour is closely linked. This denotes that attitudes may be predicted in response to certain situations. Cho and Choi (2010) note that commercial marketing often works on the assumption that a positive attitude towards a health message should result in a positive attitude towards health behaviour. What is important is the word 'should', meaning that attitudes are not always stable or consistent and therefore do not always correspond to behaviour. It is important to be clear 'about the consequences which can realistically be expected' (Downie et al., 1992) from a programme that seeks to influence or change attitudes. In health this may mean that a smoker who believes tobacco causes premature death and lung cancer may continue to smoke, or a sedentary person who believes exercise will help to lose weight remains sedentary. Because attitudes do not always correspond to behaviour they may conflict with other attitudes or go against certain social or group norms.

ACTIVITY 2.5
Attitudes and complexity

A 14-year-old five-a-day smoker may have a mixture of attitudes to cigarette smoking. On the one hand they may express positive attitudes to smoking, for example, 'I think smoking makes me look older' or 'All my friends do it, it's a social thing we do together'. On the other hand they may also express negative attitudes to smoking, for example, 'My parents don't like smoking and they don't know I smoke' or 'I don't like the smell of smoke'.

Remembering that attitudes can be contradictory and complex, and using the example above to help you, read the following sentences and list what 'attitudes' the people might have to:

1   Bowel cancer screening.
2   HIV tests.

Attitudes are made up of three aspects: cognitive, affective and conative:

- *Cognitive:* The cognitive aspect relates to the individual's evaluation of that attitude based on the knowledge, facts or information they have. For example, a person may know that taking anti-malaria tablets can prevent malaria in a high-risk zone, but they may also know other people who don't take anti-malaria tablets and have not contracted malaria. The cognitive aspect is the 'weighing-up' process of all the knowledge held about that behaviour or action.

- *Affective:* The affective aspect is the part that includes likes and dislikes, feelings or emotions. For example, a person may want to cut down their fatty food intake, but enjoys the taste of fast-food and likes the fact that it is convenient, thereby involving no preparation. The person may dislike the fact that they have put on some weight recently associated with their fast-food intake. The affective aspect is the 'weighing-up' process of likes and dislikes of the behaviour.
- *Conative:* The conative aspect is the behavioural intention towards the 'attitude' object; for example, a person may intend to avoid the gym, or a person may intend to wear a seatbelt.

THE RELATIONSHIP BETWEEN KNOWLEDGE, ATTITUDES AND BEHAVIOUR

One of the main aims of most health promotion campaigns is to increase knowledge and raise awareness of a particular health issue or topic. This is ultimately as the main goal behind campaign design (even if this is not acknowledged in the campaign itself) is usually to try and evoke a behaviour change. One model that considers the behaviour change link is the *knowledge–attitude–behaviour model*. This model is a simple linear model that postulates that with knowledge comes attitude change, and with attitude change comes behaviour change. An example of how this works using vitamin D is shown in Figure 2.3

There is some evidence to suggest that there is a causal chain between knowledge, attitude and behaviour. Marek et al. (2011) suggest that greater exposure to health information is correlated with better knowledge and more positive attitudes towards vaccinations. Tolvanen et al. (2011) note that in oral health, knowledge was shown to influence behaviour through attitudes: the importance

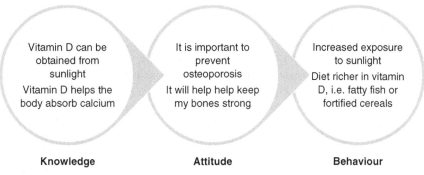

Figure 2.3   An example of the knowledge–attitude–behaviour framework

of tooth brushing for health-related reasons and better appearance being the most influential. Wong and Sam (2010) also note that in the context of information sources for pandemic influenza that those who have the most information have higher perceived susceptibility to infection. In relation to health practitioners, Roelens et al. (2006) note that education was significantly associated with screening attitude and behaviour for domestic violence.

Other studies, for example Thompson and Kumar (2011) and Lin et al. (2007), found a gap between the knowledge–attitude–behaviour relationship and the findings suggest that knowledge alone is not enough to change attitudes that lead to practising healthy behaviours. For example, Alo and Gbadebo (2011) note in Nigeria that although many respondents are aware there are health hazards to female genital cutting (FGC) prevalence rates still remain high. This might be due to the other factors that impact on decision-making, as FGC is not solely linked to individual choices but is heavily embedded in cultural values and systems. This suggests interventions may need to focus on attitudinal change acknowledging other limitations for success rather than just knowledge. Other knowledge may just be 'common' knowledge and therefore ignored, insufficient knowledge such as not knowing an amount, e.g. of alcohol, or subject to other influence that impairs judgement. For example in the UK in general all drivers are aware that drinking a large quantity of alcohol and then driving a car is illegal, yet some people still do it.

BELIEFS

>> A *belief* is a cognitive construct that is closely linked to the properties or knowledge held about an object or behaviour, i.e. believing that something is good or bad. An individual's behaviour is linked to their beliefs. Beliefs cannot be directly observed, but are often inferred based on a person's behaviour (Robinson, 2004). The individual's personal experiences inform the core beliefs that a person holds. These beliefs may be strong enough to motivate health behaviours; for example, Brown and Lee (2011) note that mothers who report ingrained and strong beliefs that they are able to overcome barriers to exclusive breastfeeding are much more likely to breastfeed. Other studies also note that positive beliefs can result in performance of that behaviour, for example medication beliefs (i.e. that it enables control of illness) predict medication adherence (Schüza et al., 2011). Beliefs can also be demonstrated through avoidance, for example beliefs in cervical cancer smear tests being intrusive or painful may result in non-attendance at screening.

In health promotion the prediction is that if someone believes something then they will perform that behaviour. For example, if a person believes that wearing reflective clothing when running at night will means cars can see them, they will wear reflective clothing. A person who believes eating fresh fruit and vegetables will decrease the risks of bowel cancer will eat fresh fruit and vegetables. Ferrante et al. (2011) note that reasons why men choose not to get prostate cancer screening include reasons such as they perceive they are at low risk due to lack of urinary symptoms, lack of family history of prostate cancer or beliefs that healthy behaviours can prevent prostate cancer. This would lead to the assumption that if these beliefs were altered men would be more likely to go for screening.

ACTIVITY 2.6
Beliefs and tobacco

Tobacco smoking is widely known to have negative health impacts yet around 30% of the population continue to smoke.

1 What do you think those that smoke tobacco believe encourages them to continue to smoke?
2 If you wanted to design a campaign to tackle these beliefs what sort of messages could you create to challenge these beliefs?

Of course, in reality it is not that simple and beliefs do not always predict or result in the performance of that behaviour, for example beliefs in the benefits of physical activity often do not result in increased uptake of physical activity. Evenson and Bradley (2010) found that pregnant women who had appropriate understanding of exercise in pregnancy and believed in benefits of physical activity for themselves and their babies were still not exercising. Nayak et al. (2010) note that older adults demonstrate several beliefs that may be barriers to osteoporosis screening such as low beliefs in susceptibility to osteoporosis, with older adults believing less strongly in osteoporosis severity than younger adults. Given that osteoporosis and the problems connected with this such as hip fractures can have a bigger impact on older adults (for example there is increased likelihood of other co-morbidities such as circulatory problems leading to lengthened healing times) this finding is important for health promotion. Similar results are found in a study examining protective behaviours during a pandemic, where those who have greater levels of perceived susceptibility and severity and greater belief in the effectiveness of recommended behaviour are more likely to perform the behaviours (Bish and Michie, 2010). There is also evidence to suggest that beliefs may be complex and difficult to identify. For example a study looking at non-adherence to medicine found that those subjects who reported 'forgetfulness and carelessness' in taking medication actually had high levels of concern beliefs about their medication (Unni and Farris, 2011) suggesting it may be hard to identify the beliefs that impact on behaviour the most.

VALUES

Values can influence attitudes by determining the importance attached to them, they 'energise' attitudes and underpin behaviour (Green and Tones, 2011). Values are usually acquired through the social world. Friends, family, society, employment or religion are all linked to values and can therefore be linked to personal or cultural values. These values can be explicit or implicit:

- *Explicit values* are those value judgements that are made and can be seen, for example, verbally discriminating against the opposite sex in a social setting.
- *Implicit values* are values that are inferred by non-verbal behaviours, for example, ignoring all members of the opposite sex in a social setting and only talking to those of the same sex.

In relation to health, the role of values suggests that a person puts a 'value' on an object or behaviour. If they regard an object or behaviour highly, for example a cigarette, then they may be more likely to smoke. If they do not value cigarettes highly they are more likely to not smoke. A person will do the same with health promotion and preventative behaviours. If a person values an aspect of health highly, such as mobility or weight loss, they are more likely to attach high importance to activities that seek to achieve those behaviours, such as regular physical activity.

APPROACHES TO CHANGING BEHAVIOUR

There are a variety of approaches to changing behaviour which can impact on attitudes, beliefs and values. Suresh (2011) suggests four approaches: strategic communication, behaviour change communication, advocacy and social mobilisation.

- *Strategic communication* is evidence-based (see Chapter 7) and undertaken with the target group tailoring information to the local context and population in order to try and elicit a change in behaviours.
- *Behaviour change communication* utilises theoretical models (see Chapter 1) and looks at segmenting audiences in order to address key issues relevant to the defined target group. A mixture of methods suitable to the audience needs are used, for example, information technology, mass media or interpersonal communication. The focus is on changing or influencing behaviour for a positive outcome.
- *Advocacy* is a process which prepares the population for acceptance of a behaviour, idea or programme at a political or social level. It accumulates information to push forward agendas and decisions and may attempt to accumulate resources in order to promote a healthy outcome, i.e. a behavioural, policy or environmental change.
- Social mobilisation brings together a multitude of different sectors to collaborate and mobilise resources to promote a climate where change can occur. Communities may identify resources they need and enlist the help of others, e.g. local groups or networks, to achieve this outcome. It is based on an empowerment model of health promotion as it facilitates a community's control of health.

The two of most interest to campaign design is strategic and behaviour change communication. As strategic communication is closely linked to healthy settings this will be covered in Chapter 7. The focus for this chapter is on behaviour change communication.

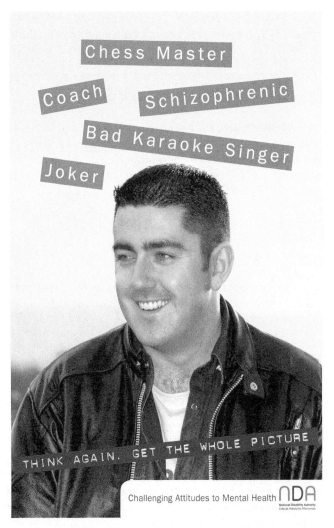

Figure 2.4 'Think again get the whole picture', poster with chess master Paul Leavy, National Disability Authority (Ireland)

It is postulated that targeting attitudes may result in a change to beliefs, values or behaviours. A good example is the poster as part of a disability campaign in Figure 2.4. The poster aims to focus on attitudes and promote attitudinal change towards mental illness by suggesting that the reader 'rethinks' or questions their own attitudes towards those with mental ill health (in this case schizophrenia), as well as illustrating that mental health does not get in the way of an active life. This is one way to challenge values and may prompt people to question what they think about mental health (i.e. the idea that those with mental illness are different or unable to live an active life). This technique has been used in a variety of campaigns to combat stigma and discrimination in relation to disability, mental health, racism and bullying. Case Study 2.1 gives an example of challenging chlamydia beliefs.

Chlamydia message design

The UK Department of Health (DH, 2008) undertook research around chlamydia before a campaign was launched in 2009–2010 to encourage chlamydia screening. Research suggested that there were widespread misconceptions about chlamydia although awareness levels of chlamydia and testing were high. They identified three main messages to focus on:

- Chlamydia is invisible.
- Chlamydia is serious.
- Chlamydia is easily spread.

Research showed that these messages individually are easily dissuaded as they were insufficient to create personal relevance. When combined with two additional strands in messages they were seen as more effective. These were:

1 Make the issue personal.
2 Make screening normal (to overcome stigma and barriers).

ACTIVITY 2.7
Designing messages to target attitudes

1 Choose a small target group and identify their age, gender, social class, ethnicity.
2 What messages could you develop using the principles in Case Study 2.1 to influence negative attitudes towards chlamydia screening?

Changing attitudes through behaviour change involves different methods from the traditional educational and information-giving approaches and is less widely used. This is partly due to cost, expertise and resource implications and can be more difficult to design, reaching a smaller number of people and sometimes requiring specialist practitioners. As Downie et al. (1992) write, you cannot paint people's skin colour to make them experience racist reactions or subject people to a nuclear winter to change attitudes to nuclear weaponry, therefore you need to utilise techniques that can imitate these scenarios. Working in small groups or with individuals face-to-face may be utilised via *role play*, experimental learning, skill teaching or other interactive methods of learning and may be part of a multi-faceted communication campaign.

Role play and experimental learning usually involve participants taking on the role of a different person in a specified setting and acting out the 'part' that person might play, either by following a script or by improvisation. For example, children might be encouraged to practise refusal skills to offers of an illegal drug or cigarettes; publicans might be encouraged to practise skills that could be used to diffuse violent incidents in pubs. One of the main purposes of role play is that people 'act' what should happen in order to then translate this into the real setting when it occurs. Experimental learning may go one step further and put people into different situations, for example, driving simulators for learner drivers giving practice that can be translated into a real situation. The Internet may offer potential advantages for this type of practice, for example a tool to simulate drinking while trying to do two things at once (DfT, 2012a).

GATEKEEPERS AND INFORMATION DISSEMINATORS

It is believed that the more people that like a communicator, the more likely people will pay attention to, and accept, the message. The use of opinion leaders in a community group may be helpful for getting a message across, particularly where there are hard-to-access groups. The two-step flow model of communication (Katz and Lazarsfeld, 1955) suggests that interpretation of media messages is a process which flows through key opinion leaders in a community. These opinion leaders gather health information and interpret, disseminate or block messages. An opinion leader can be anyone of standing or influence in a community, and can include the head of a household who has responsibility for their family health. Parents, especially mothers, are often gatekeepers to health information for older and younger family members (Koehly et al., 2009). Some studies highlight different cultural differences in gatekeepers, for example in the Hmong community in the US, group or male leaders make decisions which can impact on health outcomes (Thalacker, 2011). Mass media campaigns can also impact on those who have not seen them by interpersonal communication with people who have. Van den Putte et al. (2011) suggest a substantial number of smokers who are not directly exposed to anti-smoking campaigns are still exposed via communication to people who have seen them.

A focus on gatekeepers or opinion leaders suggests that targeting messages to them is more important than targeting messages to a target group (see Case Study 2.2). Shafer et al. (2011) demonstrates that to increase vaccination against the human papillomavirus (HPV) that causes around two-thirds of cervical cancer cases pre-testing messages with mothers of pre-teens *may be* an effective strategy rather than targeting pre-teens. For example, they found that emotional truths such as the mother's desire to protect her daughter were important and that mothers acted more positively to messages framed on preventing cervical cancer rather than preventing HPV, a sexually transmitted infection.

Gatekeepers and influential others in India

Sebastian et al. (2010) examined the promotion of health spacing between pregnancies in India. They note that in India both the husband and mother-in-law play a controlling and dominating role in female contraceptive use. Their findings suggest that many young couples want to space births but that a number of barriers limit their ability to put these desires into action. The reasons for supporting spacing vary between women, the husband and the mother-in-law. While all three groups agree that the health of the young child is the most important reason for child spacing the second reason for importance suggests three reasons. The women suggest 'their own health', the husband 'finances for child care and delivery' and the mother-in-law 'household expenses'. Audience-specific messages were developed for the three groups based on their prioritisation.

IMPLICATIONS FOR PRACTICE

In order to design effective strategies for diverse audiences it is important to understand the similarities and differences between groups. As social and psychological factors are intertwined the relationship between the separate components are difficult to separate out and may all impact on practice. Case Study 2.3 is an example of childhood obesity and the recommendations for prevention and treatment which include a mix of social, psychological and other factors addressed in different sections of this textbook.

Influential factors in the prevention of obesity

Caprio et al. (2008) publish a list of consensus recommendations for the prevention and treatment of childhood obesity. Below are some adapted recommendations. Note the relationships between the wide range of factors:

- Children should be viewed in the context of their families, communities and cultures.
- Obesity risk discussion should take into account the education level and socioeconomic status of children/families.
- Breastfeeding should be encouraged.
- Restriction of youth-targeted television advertising of foods with low nutritional value.
- Consider cultural, individual, gender, family preferences and realities of time and money with regard to advice about meal planning and physical activity.

There are a variety of aspects to remember in relation to social and psychological factors when designing health promotion campaigns. First, you need to know everything you can that is relevant about your target audience. Map out their social and psychological characteristics in relation to age, gender, social group, education levels and culture alongside attitudes, beliefs, values and other variables that might be important in a campaign. Your chosen theoretical model may give you some ideas about additional variables, for example perceived behavioural control, subjective norm or benefits and barriers. Ask the target group what information preference they have. Research is limited in this area that can be widely applied to different groups, and with the growth of new technologies (e.g. the Internet or mobile phones) preferences for information will change.

Collaborate with representatives from the population in the design of materials. Include the target group in the design of the programme, as they will be able to identify important factors that are essential in health behaviours. For example a study that designed a brief web-based alcohol intervention in college students collected qualitative data that examined various aspects of drinking behaviour and the drinking culture (e.g. attitudes towards alcohol use; when, where and why drinking occurred [Barretto et al., 2010]). Engage key organisations and groups that the target group utilises or works closely with, and work with gatekeepers or key opinion leaders of different groups; for example, consider the use of wider resources for some groups, such as interpreters for different language groups or the use of youth workers for young people.

When working with different ethnic or cultural groups and lower education levels, educational materials should be adapted to different needs. Consider different ways of imparting information to these groups (see Chapters 4 and 5). Develop, design and distribute accurate information in a culturally sensitive and appropriate way.

Finally, choose your theoretical model and methods carefully. Different theoretical models emphasise areas that might be more relevant to your target group, setting or behaviour. You will also need to select your method according to what you are trying to achieve. One method will not suit all. Corcoran (2011) has a list of questions that will be helpful to consider when working with target groups.

CONCLUSION

Current research has *underutilised* the role of the target group in the development and design of communication strategies to the detriment of these campaigns, particularly in non-Western populations and hard-to-reach groups. Future research should also consider sub-populations in groups.

A good health communication strategy will have a rationale that is based on a clearly identified target group in terms of both social and psychological factors. Health promotion should plan, implement and evaluate information in a way that allows the desired audience to take in information, digest this and then implement it immediately or at a later date as appropriate. By identifying the social and psychological factors of a group and matching their preferences to information, the outcome is more likely to be relevant, achievable and successful.

Summary

- This chapter has examined the role of the target group and their own characteristics in health promotion communication design.
- The social factors of age, sex, social class, education, ethnicity, culture and religion, alongside the psychological factors of attitudes, beliefs and values have been examined and their links to the target group demonstrated.
- Strategies for changing attitudes with particular reference to knowledge and design of campaigns has been considered.

ADDITIONAL READING

This book has a chapter on practically working with target groups and their social and psychological factors: Corcoran N (2011) *Working on Health Communication*. Sage, London.

A good article to illustrate the relationships between social variables: Caprio S, Daniels SR, Drewnowski A, Kaufman FR, Palinkas LA, Rosenbloom AL and Schwimmer JB (2008) Influence of race, ethnicity and culture on childhood obesity: Implications for prevention and treatment. *Diabetes Care* 31 (11): 2211–2220.

3

REACHING UNREACHABLE GROUPS AND CROSSING CULTURAL BARRIERS

CALVIN MOORLEY, BARBARA GOODFELLOW AND NOVA CORCORAN

Learning objectives:

- Explain the cultural barriers that exist in relation to communication in health settings and consider ways in which these might be overcome.
- Identify the issues around communicating in health settings with different cultural groups, people living with disabilities and older people and consider ways in which these might be overcome.
- Identify the barriers to communicating health to different cultural groups, people living with disabilities and older people and the implications for practice.

The term 'hard-to-reach groups' may be used to describe a wide range of individuals and groups of people and may in itself be contested. The term might infer blame and lead in turn to prejudice or *discrimination*. Nevertheless, it is currently recognised that in the UK there are many sections of our society who are, or feel themselves to be, living on the margins of the mainstream. Politically this status has been recognised and the term 'socially excluded' has been applied to these and many other groups to whom the following discussion is relevant. The specific groups that have been selected for discussion in this chapter are: people from ethnic minority cultures, people living with long-term disability and older people. Issues or difficulties around communication and health are common to them all. What is clear is that in order to deliver, develop or design health care of the best possible standard to these, often high-need groups, good communication between them and the service providers is essential.

The NHS of the twenty-first century must be responsive to the needs of different groups and individuals within society, and challenge discrimination on the grounds of age, gender, ethnicity, religion, disability and sexuality. People with communication disabilities are at risk of not being able to communicate effectively with their health care providers. This could mean directly compromising their health, health care and their individual right to participate actively in decisions about their health care (O'Halloran et al., 2008). Communication difficulties are apparent in a range of hard-to-reach groups and this chapter will consider culture, physical disabilities and older people in the exploration of these issues.

CROSSING CULTURAL BARRIERS

The concepts of culture and ethnicity

Although no single definition of culture is accepted by social scientists, it is generally agreed that culture is learned, shared and transmitted from one generation to another. Culture is reflected in a group's values, norms, practices, system of meaning (including language and communication) and way of life. The concept of ethnicity is more problematic but is usually used to denote groups of people who share similar histories which give them a distinct identity to a homeland (Robinson, 2002). As highlighted in Chapter 2 ethnicity is a term used to categorise groups based on cultural characteristics such as shared ancestry, religion or language. Race is a term used to distinguish biologically between groups. Culture can reflect both of these concepts and is a 'system of shared understanding that shapes and, in turn, is shaped by experience' (Caprio et al., 2008: 2214).

ACTIVITY 3.1
Cultural identity

1 Consider what you think of as your cultural identity.
2 How do you think it impacts (or could impact) on you as a health practitioner in your communication and interaction with others?
3 Consider ways in which ethnicity and culture impacts on the lives of individuals you may come into contact with as a health practitioner.

Distribution and needs of different groups

The latest census recorded that of the UK population in 2001 the majority were white (92.1%) (ONS, 2001). The remaining 4.6 million (or 7.9%) belonged to other ethnic groups. Indians were the largest of these groups, followed by Pakistanis, those of mixed ethnic background, Black Caribbeans, Black Africans and Bangladeshis (ONS, 2001). The same data show that people from minority groups were more likely than white people to live in low income households. Generally data show that immigrant groups have worse health outcomes than the majority population and are vulnerable to serious health disparities and higher rates of morbidity and mortality (Kreps and Sparks, 2008). As well as differences in self-assessed general health, men and women varied in their likelihood of having specific diseases. One area where this was particularly marked was in the prevalence of self-reported diabetes. Such findings further confirm the importance of addressing communication between health care providers and minority health care users, especially those who lack fluency in English. Communication interventions to educate vulnerable populations need to be strategic and evidence-based. It is important for health educators to adopt culturally sensitive communication practices to reach and influence vulnerable populations (Kreps and Sparks, 2008).

Strategies for enhancing cultural awareness

Kreuter et al. (2002, 2003) suggest that health programmes and health promotion programmes in particular should make explicit attempts to develop culturally appropriate strategies to meet the needs of special populations. The authors state that health professionals must be able to identify and describe cultures within a given population and understand how each relates to health beliefs and actions. One of the strategies put forward is that of culturally tailored communication, which can be described as any combination of information or change strategy intended to reach one particular person. This can be contrasted with targeting, which is directed towards groups rather than individuals. There is clearly a paradox here in that culture is a shared group characteristic, so if something is not shared can it be cultural?

One of the most common ways of increasing participation of different cultural groups in health promotion interventions is the adaptation of existing health promotion programmes for different cultural groups. This requires understanding of the cultural beliefs and values, traditions, lifestyles and philosophies of the group in question. For example Leake et al. (2011) note that to increase attendance in a lifestyle intervention for Filipino-American participants inclusion of activities, foods and proverbs consistent with Filipino culture were important. Kulukulualani et al. (2008) in their development of culturally tailored cancer brochures with native Hawaiians noted that family associations were important, and the target group wanted materials that incorporated traditional Hawaiian values. These included notions of the family, being part of a group and the natural environment. See Case Study 3.1 for an example of cultural differences.

Kreuter et al. (2003) suggest a range of culturally specific planning strategies for campaigns ranging from minimal intervention titled 'peripheral' (adapting existing materials to ensure they are culturally appropriate) to 'sociocultural' (in which cultural aspects of the audience are located in the context of the wider social context) (see Corcoran, 2011). A good way of targeting individuals rather than the group would be to employ workers from within the group (a 'constituent involving' strategy according to Kreuter et al., 2003). In such cases the health worker would have insider knowledge of how the group thinks and operates thus making it easier to set targets and communicate health. Buchthal et al. (2011) suggest that cultural tailoring may not be enough to reach all ethnic minority groups especially those in low income groups, suggesting use of constituent involving strategies or sociocultural strategies may be more effective.

Case Study 3.1

Trachoma control programmes and cultural differences

The SAFE strategy for trachoma control was evaluated in eight countries worldwide. SAFE is an acronym for the action that is needed to implement a trachoma control strategy:

S – Strategy explaining the disease process and need for trichiasis surgery.

A – Mass antibiotic distribution and acceptance of antibiotics.

F – Facial cleanliness/hygiene promotion.

E – Environmental changes, such as building and using latrines.

Evaluation of the programmes in these eight countries found that different methods were used in different countries to promote similar SAFE messages. Community meetings were seen as a good place to discuss trachoma, and were conducted in a variety of church, mosque, club or society settings. Where local cultural norms were ignored or where providers failed to approach communities in an appropriate manner, there was some resistance to the programme.

The SAFE message was transmitted via different settings in different countries, including schools-based programmes, mass media messages from different media (television, radio) and in different formats including songs and drama. Health centres and clinics and one-to-one work were also found effective in some locations. Locally based communicators were also seen as important as they are known to their peer groups. (Zondervan et al., 2004)

COMMUNICATING ACROSS CULTURAL BARRIERS

There is a growing realisation of the extent of cultural and language variation among ethnic minority users of health and social services. This has great significance for countries such as England who have become a home for migrant workers and those seeking refuge. Despite policy initiatives, empirical studies provide evidence that on an individual face-to-face level the communication needs of ethnic minority groups are not always being effectively met. In addition research in the growing area of online communication may not be meeting diverse audience needs. For example Neuhauser and Kreps (2008) note that online cancer communication has not met the literacy, cultural and linguistic needs of diverse populations.

Communication difficulties in caring for people from ethnic minority groups, especially those not fluent in English, may be seen as obstacles to the provision of health services and care. For example health practitioners of different cultural backgrounds may not always understand the culture of their patients. In the US Clayman et al. (2010) found that those Hispanics/Latinos who were comfortable speaking English had higher media exposure and higher trust of health information from newspapers, magazines and the Internet. This suggests those who find it more difficult to speak the dominant language may access media less and have lower trust in media sources. Language is a key component of acculturation and is often measured by English ability. Evidence suggests for example in smoking cessation that Latinos with low acculturation use NRT (nicotine replacement therapy) less often than non-Latino whites residing in that area. Similar results have been found for mammography use (Liang et al., 2009). This highlights a possible lack of information about health and access to health care resources and an absence of culturally sensitive and language appropriate health promotion materials.

ACTIVITY 3.2
Barriers to health

1 Identify the barriers that those from different cultural groups may experience in terms of accessing health services.
2 If you were designing a health campaign that aimed to increase access to cancer screening services how would you address these barriers in a health campaign? Think about the wording, images or other communication tools you might use.

There are a number of other barriers to health promotion. For example, in research around female groups it has been proposed that non-English-speaking women may not receive adequate maternity care unless their needs are met via interpreters or advocates (Rowe and Garcia, 2003). Jacobs et al. (2005) also found that women who spoke little or no English in an English-speaking country were less likely to receive screening for breast and cervical cancers, particularly cervical cancer. In a health promotion context this may mean the provision of preventative services, or preventative messages, is unable to be transmitted unless adequate alternatives are sought. Moorley (2010) found that Afro-Caribbean women living with stroke held cultural beliefs that disease (in this case stroke and resulting disability) impacts on the way women are perceived culturally.

Another instance of a process barrier to communication is cited by Vydelingum (2000), who studied a small number of hospital patients and carers in a mixed ethnic minority group. This study found that language barriers and communication difficulties which accompanied this led to feelings of extreme isolation. Vydelingum observed that these communication difficulties were exacerbated by other factors, including lack of positive action on the part of the nurses in providing resources to aid effective communication, and that nurses were perceived as too busy to respond to patients' needs. Another factor which might also hinder good communication is the application of caring models in which there is a high expectation of patient involvement, which may not be fully appreciated by the patient or their family and would not be the norm in their culture. Stereotyping may also further compound poor communication.

STRUCTURAL BARRIERS

In the UK it is not acceptable that environmental barriers inhibit access to health care. Evidence, however, suggests that these structural barriers are still in place. Robinson (2002) notes a number of areas that need to be considered in relation to the way in which organisational aspects undermine the quality of communication and care. He states: 'in the area of assessment of minority ethnic user needs by community consultation, gathering and use of information about individual patients' communication needs, bilingual support, practitioner education, and provision of material resources, organizational shortcomings have been demonstrated' (Robinson, 2002: 15). O'Halloran et al. (2008) also suggest a number of environmental barriers inhibiting access to services in people with communication difficulties.

Case Study 3.2

Black and Afro-Caribbean groups and mental health

Baker and Macpherson (2000) found that black and Afro-Caribbean people are more likely to:

- Be diagnosed with schizophrenia.
- Receive physical treatment when in care.
- Not receive counselling or psychotherapy or see black counsellors.
- Be regarded as violent, located in locked wards and have longer stays in medium secure care.
- Receive higher doses of medication.
- Find their way into hospital via the police, compulsory admission under the Mental Health Act or from prison.
- Overall, black people have poorer outcomes after care. (Fernando, 2003; Wallcraft, 2003)

ACTIVITY 3.3
Challenging the present

1 Consider the list in Case Study 3.2 and think about how many items on this list involve communication between the service user and service provider.
2 If you were working with a black or Afro-Caribbean group in the community, how might you try to reduce any of these variables via health promotion practice?

Reasons given to explain why black people and others from ethnic minority backgrounds appear to have higher rates of mental illness and a different, often coercive relationship with services include: racist and prejudiced attitudes on the part of service providers and agencies of the state, such as the police; a lack of cultural sensitivity; more frequent exposure to stressors such as unemployment; and adjusting to a new society. It is clear that for many aspects of the NHS modernisation agenda to work in reality requires a shift in the balance of power, which must be supported by a real culture change in the way services are provided and particularly in the way in which communication takes place between service providers and users from ethnic minority groups. See also Case Study 3.2.

COMMUNICATION AND PEOPLE LIVING WITH DISABILITIES

It is estimated that there are around 650 million disabled people worldwide (World Bank, 2012), the largest number of whom are to be found in high income countries. However, there is a higher prevalence of disabled people relative to population numbers in the low income countries. It is clear that with advances in medicine which prolong life and the demographic changes in the age of the population these numbers will increase. There are many types of disability, including sensory and learning disability. For the purpose of this textbook the emphasis will be on people living with physical disability. People living with disabilities face a series of problems in relation to their communication needs and often assumed difficulties are addressed, for example with hearing or speech, but they may not always be addressed by alternative communication methods. For example Zazove et al. (2012) note that deaf persons have a poorer understanding of cancer prevention, which is felt to be partly due to communication barriers. They designed a video adapted for a deaf population with culture-specific communications (i.e. American Sign Language, captions) but found it had no increase on cancer knowledge. Yao et al. (2012) developed a cervical screening video with similar adaptations but screened this to both a hearing and deaf population and found that although both groups increase knowledge, the hearing women's score were higher. These examples illustrate the problematic nature of communication and the assumptions that health professionals may make but that still may not go far enough to ensure effective communication.

THE CLASSIFICATION AND DEFINITION OF DISABILITY

The classical way to view disability is to see it as a medical problem. It is this approach that is the basis for most current health and social policy, and also that which lies at the centre of much medical treatment aimed at people with disabilities. It is the basis of the World Health Organization's (WHO, 2000) International Classification of Impairments, Disabilities and Handicaps (ICIDH). This approach assumes that impairments are the result of biological or psychological abnormality, and that disabilities are the resulting barriers to activity and handicaps are the disadvantages faced by people with disabilities as a result of this.

Such classification locates 'the problem' with the individual and provides a deficit model of disability where people with disabilities are viewed as powerless objects of policy rather than as citizens. From 1960 onwards large numbers of disabled people felt that traditional politics had failed them and there was a shift in the way they were managed and treated, with an emphasis on user organisation and self-reliance with a political rather than medical orientation. This shift was also underpinned by the adoption of a social rather than a medical model of health.

LABELLING AND STIGMA

Language is critical in shaping our thoughts, beliefs, values and attitudes. Some words by their very nature degrade and diminish people with a disability. The language customarily used to denote disability has been condemnatory, and perhaps the most dangerous use of language in describing a person with a disability has been to dehumanise the individual by labelling the person as the disability. In the past people with disabilities have been stigmatised. 'Labelling' and 'stigma' are terms used to describe negative evaluations of individuals or groups by other individuals or groups. The terms are important for health workers because their ability consciously or unconsciously to apply such labels to people with disabilities reflects the traditional power held by such workers, especially practitioners in the medical profession. Angermeyer et al. (2009) note the increase in campaigns that aim to address mental health stigma but suggest in a review that while there was an increase in the mental health literacy of the public, the desire for social distance from people with major depression and schizophrenia remains the same and that educating people against mental disorders does not automatically reduce stigma.

This is problematic as this strategy remains a popular way to address stigma in mental health. (See, for example, Figure 2.4 in Chapter 2.)

ACTIVITY 3.4
Disability campaigns

Have a look at the following websites and their campaigns to address disability related issues:

- Mencap (2012) and their campaign to end hate crime available at www.mencap.org. uk/standbyme.
- Centre for Chronic Disease Prevention and Health Promotion's (CDC) (2009, 2012) Right to Know campaign for breast screening available at www.cdc.gov/ ncbddd/disabilityandhealth/righttoknow/.

1 What are the predominant methods that are used in these campaigns?
2 What are the main aims of these campaigns?
3 Do you think these are effective?
4 If you were working on a health campaign in either of these areas what else could you do?

HEALTH PROMOTION – COMMUNICATION AND LANGUAGE

Thompson (2002) observes that health practitioners who are working with disabled people need to recognise the social roots of disability and stigma so that they can avoid:

- Allowing negative stereotypes to mar interpersonal interactions;
- Reinforcing or exacerbating the social disadvantages associated with disability; and
- Disempowering disabled people.

Health practitioners need to be sensitive to the fact that disability acts as a form of social oppression, and practice therefore needs to be geared towards challenging such oppression rather than reinforcing it. The potential of communication and particularly language to reinforce or exacerbate oppression is often not fully recognised. We need to realise that language not only reflects reality but also contributes to creating and maintaining that reality. Language can transmit the dominant ideas that perpetuate inequality and disadvantage for people with disabilities. Figure 3.1 illustrates the notion that discrimination in society is reflected in language, and in turn language reinforces discrimination in society.

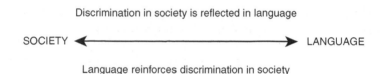

Figure 3.1   The double standard of language and disability

HEALTH CARE COMMUNICATION AND DISABILITY

People with disability, and their families, typically have frequent and ongoing communication with a wide variety of health and social care professionals, depending on the nature and severity of their condition. Research by Lindsay et al. (2012) notes five areas where immigrant parents caring for children with a disability encounter challenges in health and community care. These are lack of training in providing culturally sensitive care, language and communication issues, discrepancies in conceptualisations of disability between health care providers and immigrant parents, building rapport and helping parents to advocate for themselves and their children. This suggests that health communication has a number of possible starting points to work from to improve health outcomes.

There is considerable evidence to indicate that patient satisfaction is closely related to the communication skills of health care workers. However, professional communication is an area in which health care provision often does not meet patient needs. Such professional communication might be that with nurses, physiotherapists, occupational therapists and other allied health professionals. Prominent among the health care relationships that have been the subject of previous research is that of the doctor–patient relationship, and while this is recognised as remaining significant there is now increasing attention being drawn to a wider patient experience. Health practitioners should be continually developing new ways to communicate with disabled people. New information technology (IT) such as *smart phones* and *tablets* can be used to aid communication with disabled people by using different applications. This also means that there is an onus on the health practitioner to update their own knowledge on using information communication (see Chapter 5 for more on IT).

DEFINING, PROFILING AND LOCATING OLDER PEOPLE

One of the concerns of health promotion is reaching different groups, and identifying these groups can prove difficult and should be done with great accuracy. The definition of the group labelled as 'older people' has had some differing opinions across the world (Tinker, 1997). In the UK the term 'older people' usually refers to those over retirement age; in the US the term 'elders' is used to describe the same group. Tomassini (2005) has highlighted that studies focusing on older people have formulated categories of ageing. These are the 'young old' aged between 65 and 74 years, the 'old old' aged between 75 and 90 years and the 'very old', over 90 years. The 2001 census in the UK confirmed what most people who work with older people thought: that in the UK we have a growing older population. In the UK there are over 10.3 million people aged 65 and over. The number of people aged 65 and over is also predicted to increase. Projections suggest 12.7 million in 2018 and 16.9 million by 2035 (House of Commons, 2012) reveals that in 2003 there were over 20 million people aged 50 and over resident in the UK.

Ageing is an interesting phenomenon, as being 'old' is often viewed in a biological and social context. The age of an individual is a chronological event, therefore measured in years. More frequently age is measured in abilities, beginning with the young – when a child starts walking or talking – or in other words, through physical and cognitive development. For older adults ageing tends to be measured mainly in terms of physical and psychological deteriorations. There are three main approaches to defining ageing. First the chronological approach, which looks at the age of the individual in terms of number of years lived. The second approach is based on subjective perception. It takes into account how the individual feels, what their age means to them, and also social meanings of their age. The final approach is linked to social construction, where the social representation of age in institutions (such as hospitals, prisons, universities, colleges) and government departments' ideologies and structural interest determine age. For example, some companies may have different policies on the age of retirement, which may not always be in agreement with national guidelines. Some educational institutions may label their students according to their age, for example students over 21 years in the UK are commonly referred to as 'mature' students. These variations of age are important to bear in mind when designing health promotion work, as a health practitioner will have to consider what sort of 'age' will be used in their work.

The study of ageing and older people falls under the discipline of gerontology and is viewed as a multidisciplinary approach to the study of ageing; rather than a pure science, it draws from the social and physical sciences (Jamieson, 2002). This multidisciplinary approach can lead to different emphasis on the health and quality of life of older people. While the physical science may focus on the functional ability of older people, the social science may choose to concentrate on the meaning and value of experiences of ageing. Both are of equal importance to health promoters and planners in meeting the needs of this target group. Another important consideration is how older people themselves view their health. Blaxter (1990, 1997) noted in her study that as we grow older emphasis on what it is to be healthy changes. For example in later life financial security and ability to function becomes more important to older people.

Older people, though visible within society, can be difficult to locate, mainly due to the macro (structural and societal) and individual (personal) perspectives. Moorley (2012) found that in life after stroke research conducted on an inner city Afro-Caribbean population that participants saw ageing as being influenced by the societal, cultural economic and political context prevailing in their everyday life which led to changes in the behaviour and attitude of participants. This suggests that the wider needs of older people may go unrecognised despite the wider societal environment remaining a strong influence in health and health care.

HEALTH AND WELLBEING

The ageing process in the UK has been reported as a time of negative decline which exposes individuals to increasing risk of illness and disability. Health is an important concern for older people; it is a period of life where the ability to maintain good health is seen as the key to remaining independent, allowing them to perform normal daily activities. For older people health may mean different things. For example it may mean the ability to be physically independent, to be able to get from one place to another, which includes driving and the feeling of safety while doing so. It may mean to be financially independent, to be able to make independent choices and not be instructed on what to do but given the freedom of choice, or to be able to have a social network that they can rely on. Hughner and Kleine (2004) sought to understand how lay people think about health and its meaning and place in their daily lives. Their older participants defined health as the ability to function and do things while for younger participants health was more to do with physical and mental wellbeing and self-realisation. This has an important role in the framing of health messages and the motivations of people to be involved in health campaigns. It is also important that health practitioners acknowledge the subjective definitions of health and build them into the structural/macro concepts of ageing in order to communicate effective health messages to older people.

The Age UK website

Age UK, the largest organisation in the UK working with and for older people, has a website with information designed specifically for older people. It contains a wealth of information including policy documentation and key issues. It also contains health and lifestyle information including advice around exercise, healthy eating, relationships and health care rights alongside finance, work and learning.

To try and facilitate access to their website for those who might have 'accessibility' problems they include a 'display options' function to change colour and font size, and information on how to navigate the website without using a mouse. (www.ageuk.org.uk/)

COMMUNICATION AND BARRIERS TO WORKING WITH OLDER PEOPLE

The world's population is ageing; in the UK we are now experiencing a low demographic regime (or in other words, a low fertility rate) and a growing larger, older population. There are rapid changes to the lives of older people influenced by advanced technology and economic and social developments. Such developments can produce many challenges to providing good quality care to older people. This means that communication disorders that may limit mobility, vision, endurance or cognition will become more prevalent (Yorkston et al., 2010). An additional effect is that older people will become the largest consumer group of health and health care provisions. In order to address these needs competently, we need to be able to communicate effectively to the targeted audience on a group and individual level. For example Sparks and Nussbaum (2008) note that older adults who are diagnosed with cancer must confront a health care system that demands a high level of health literacy to successfully manage the disease. This may mean that they are at a distinct disadvantage in their ability to successfully cope with cancer because of age-related physiological, cognitive, psychological and communicative factors. Case Study 3.4 has an example of website accessibility ideas.

As detailed in Chapter 1, communication between individuals and groups is a complex process of 'interaction' whereby there is a sender, a message (through a mode of transmission) and a receiver. In order for communication to occur, the sender must be clear on what message they want to send, choose the appropriate mode of transmission and ensure that the receiver gets the message as it was originally sent or intended. Knowledge of communication skills is important and can enhance the communication process when communicating health to older people. In order to make full use of verbal and non-verbal communication skills, the health care worker and those concerned with the older person need to have an awareness of the possible barriers to communicating with the group or individual. These barriers can be divided into two categories, arising mainly from the biological (physical) and the psychosocial components of the ageing process.

Due to the changes in physical cell activity (biological), the effect of ageing pathology on the central nervous system can lead to physical decline. Figure 3.2 illustrates the problems and possible solutions to improving communication in groups that may have visual, hearing or speech impairment. Health communication may be more difficult, and may require materials or content to be adapted accordingly.

Figure 3.2 identifies some of the areas that should be considered when communicating messages with an older age group. Many of these may be seen as common sense, for example maintaining eye contact, but these actions can make the difference between comprehension and lack of comprehension of a message. The assistance of additional health professionals such as occupational therapists, speech and language therapists or physiotherapists may be invaluable in your work with different groups within the older age range, especially if the older person is experiencing cognitive impairment. Multidisciplinary working is essential for effective communication with older age groups.

ACTIVITY 3.5
'Stop smoking' materials for those over 70

You are working for a 'stop smoking' service and you have been asked to design some stop smoking information for a group of individuals over 70, some of whom have sight impairments. Based on Figure 3.2:

1 What might you include in the design of your materials?
2 Would you be able to design one resource that would be suitable for everyone?

Problem	Style of communication	Ways to maximise communication
Visual impairment	Face-to-face/group	• Direct eye contact • Ensure glasses are clean and the correct pair
	Media-based	• Use large font materials • Use aids such as large print literature, talking books, audio materials • Use the enlarged screen setting for electronic communication
	Other points	• Maintain familiar environment to reduce risk of accidents
Hearing impairment	Face-to-face/group	• Face the person(s) so that they are able to lip read • Speak slowly and clearly • Use questions and answers to check understanding
	Media-based	• Use communication to enhance the spoken word, e.g. pictures and writing, subtitled audio-visual material, electronic communication (e.g. email)
	Other points	• Eliminate background noise • Ensure hearing aids are working and switched on
Speech	Face-to-face/group	• Speak slowly and clearly using simple sentences • Allow time for the person to respond • Encourage the use of gestures, nodding, blinking, thumbs up, etc.
	Media-based	• Choose aids such as pictures, cue cards, written instructions, IT-based programmes (e.g. email, chat rooms)
	Other points	• Observe signs of non-verbal communication (e.g. distress)

Figure 3.2 Ways to overcome visual, speech or hearing difficulties, adapted from Marr and Kershaw (1998)

The other challenges that could be encountered in working with older people include psychosocial barriers. These may exist due to an older individual withdrawing from society (see the disengagement theory discussed earlier), the loss of family or partner, loss of income, moving home to a smaller dwelling, or due to financial difficulties alongside the impact of physical or neurodegenerative disorders. Communication with older people who are cognitively impaired should be undertaken by those who are professionally trained to work with such people, as cognitive impairment can result in memory loss, disorientation, confusion, wandering and problems in recognising family members and friends.

ACTIVITY 3.6
'Healthy heart' programme design

You are working for a local hospital and you are running a 'Healthy heart' class for the over-sixties. Participants are given a variety of options to try to reduce their risk of coronary heart disease, including light physical activity and healthy eating classes. You want to encourage individuals to attend who have been identified as high risk. These individuals have been sent invitations in the post but so far have not attended, and you suspect this is because they do not want to join a group.

1 What might you do to encourage people to attend?
2 What messages other than 'health' messages could encourage people to attend?
3 What other options could be provided for people who do not want to join a group (apart from meeting people face-to-face)?

OLDER PEOPLE'S HEALTH POLICY AND HEALTH PROMOTION

The recent improvements in care and health services for older people in England have been largely influenced by the *National Service Framework for Older People* (DH, 2001), which advocates eight set standards involving the care of older people (see Figure 3.3).

The NSF eight standards for older people are:
• Rooting out age discrimination
• Person-centred care
• Intermediate care
• General hospital care
• Stroke
• Falls
• Mental health in older people
• The promotion of health and active life in older people

Figure 3.3 *The National Service Framework for Older People* (DH, 2001)

This Framework is the first ever comprehensive strategy to ensure fair, high-quality, integrated health and social care services for older people. It is a 10-year programme of action linking services to support independence and promote good health, specialised services for key conditions and culture change so that all older people and their carers are always treated with respect, dignity and fairness (DH, 2001).

>>

ACTIVITY 3.7
National Service Framework demonstrated outcomes

The *National Service Framework (NSF) for Older People* indicates that local health systems have to demonstrate each year improvements in:

- Flu immunisation.
- Smoking cessation.
- Blood pressure management.

If you were designing a campaign to increase uptake of services available in one of these three areas:

1   What methods do you think might be appropriate?
2   What key messages might you give that are appropriate for older people?

It is important to acknowledge that this Framework uses the goals of health and social policy to benefit older people. It allows the promotion of health to extend a healthy active life and at the same time trying to compress morbidity. The compression of morbidity is seen as the period of life before death spent in frailty and dependency (DH, 2001). The Framework allows health and social care workers to identify emerging problems ahead of crisis and thus reduce long-term dependency. Through the use of this Framework it is easier to anticipate and respond to problems, recognising the complex interaction of physical, mental and social care factors that may compromise independence and quality of life in older people. This

>> Framework is all-encompassing and enables planning to include global and *holistic* concepts when designing care for older people. When planning interventions for older people, this policy document is essential in setting targets, specifying target areas and providing guidelines to health promotion work.

ACTIVITY 3.8
Older people and sexual health

One area of older people's health that has not been paid much attention is their sexual health. There are increases in older people (50+) living with HIV/AIDS. The sexual health of older people is not acknowledged in health policy nor are there any directives on reporting of HIV and AIDS among older people in Europe.

1 How would you approach the topic of sexuality and health among older people?
2 Can you identify reasons why there is an increase in older people with sexually transmitted infections?

One of the challenges for health promotion in older people is to identify the opportunities in old age for improving health. To achieve this effectively we need to take account of differences and changes in lifestyle and the impact of cultural and religious beliefs. Cultural and religious beliefs can be accommodated in local health strategies that specifically promote healthy ageing for the selected client group. When planning local health promotion activities for older people it must be acknowledged that older people are not homogeneous but are a diverse group, in terms of health and fitness, dependency, socioeconomic status, levels of social exclusion and ethnicity. Chapter 2 discusses social and psychological factors of target groups in more detail. As health practitioner and promoter you will need to acknowledge that older people from different regions of a country will have different health needs. With older people and health care one size does not fit all.

CONCLUSION

As part of a health task force, we need to assess continually how we can reach individuals and groups in order to deliver health promotion. To achieve this goal health practitioners will need to be objective, with a level of sensitivity that will allow them to reach a group that can often be hidden within the wider community. The first step starts with listening. There needs to be greater consultation with groups: different cultural groups, people living with disabilities and older people. These include the people themselves, networks and advocates in order to be able to assess their health promotion needs. Always ask the target group what they want before planning an intervention. The second stage needs to assess current legislation and look at the different ways that these groups can become more inclusive in local policy and health agendas. Finally, the strategies used in health promotion need to reflect the time and place the targeted group lives in.

New technology may go some way towards meeting health needs, for example, the use of computers and mobile phones can be useful in helping older people to better understand health and meet their own health needs. This could include *SMS messaging* or email for GP appointments. Another example can be creating online *chat rooms* about issues identified by target groups, for example, different cultural groups. This can be moderated for and by the target group with the assistance of health professionals, and is a simple way of targeting this group. By allowing people to participate in the setting up of the system, we are using the participatory approach with an emancipatory goal. In reaching these hard-to-reach groups we not only impart health but also learn, and it is this symbiotic relationship that allows us to work in harmony.

Summary

- This chapter has explored the role of health promotion and health care in relation to cultural groups, people living with disabilities and older people.
- It has identified issues around communicating with these groups, alongside highlighting barriers to communication with these groups.
- This chapter has explored strategies and solutions to overcoming these barriers to enable health promotion communication in these hard-to-reach groups.

ADDITIONAL READING

For a variety of views around mental health and ethnicity try Fernando S and Keating F (2008) *Mental Health in a Multi-ethnic Society: A multidisciplinary handbook*. Routledge, London.

A practical view of ageing and health is Harwood J (2007) *Understanding Communication and Aging: Developing knowledge and awareness*. Sage, London.

Part of the Routledge Communication Series, this book has some good links to ethnicity: Ellis DG (2011) *Crafting Society: Ethnicity, class, and communication theory*. Routledge, London.

4

MASS MEDIA

NOVA CORCORAN

Learning objectives:

- Analyse the role of mass media in health promotion programmes and campaigns.
- Explore the design of mass media campaigns utilising best practice and the principles of social marketing for health promotion.
- Examine current debates in the use of media and exploring the alternative roles of media in health promotion contexts.

The use of mass media in health has been strongly linked to the achievement of health promotion aims and continues to be an attractive way to promote health to the wider population. In a health promotion context mass media are most frequently used to provide information across a range of health topics alongside attempts to promote behaviour change. Mass media are also used to advocate social, political and environmental change as well as prompt audiences to engage in dialogue about their own health. This chapter will examine the role of mass media in health promotion and discuss effective strategies for using mass media. Alternative ways of utilising the media in health promotion will be explored, including techniques for creating messages, social marketing principles, branding and media advocacy.

WHAT IS MASS MEDIA?

Mass media have an important social, economic and political role in society. It is difficult to imagine a world without mass media, as they provide a constant backdrop to the societies in which we live and influence the decisions that we make in life. Daily we are on the receiving end of a multitude of media messages and we live in an increasingly 'fractured and cluttered' (Wakefield et al., 2010: 1268) globalised media world. Health practitioners need to strive to design innovative messages that can be heard above other media messages, many of which promote unhealthy behaviours and choices. 'Mass media plays [sic] several important functions in society, including providing information, entertainment, articulating and creating meaning, setting agendas for individual and societal discourse and influencing behaviour' (Grilli et al., 2006: 2). As a health practitioner, the use of mass media in relation to health communication is of particular importance because it remains widely used in conjunction with the principles of health promotion. One of the roles of a health practitioner is to communicate health information in an accurate, timely and appropriate manner and this act often utilises media sources.

The mass media as a tool to promote health have been utilised extensively (Noar, 2006) and research suggests that mass media campaigns can be successful (see Wakefield et al., 2010). Mass media prove a popular choice of method in health promotion for their potential to modify knowledge, attitudes and some aspects of behaviour. For example there is evidence to suggest that mass media campaigns can prevent the uptake of smoking in young people although the evidence is not strong (Brinn et al., 2010). A number of studies recommend the use of media campaigns to change health behaviours (see, for example, Vallone et al., 2011) and it has been suggested that mass media campaigns can influence a variety of lifestyle-related behaviours, for example physical activity (Webb et al., 2011). Synder (2007) considers that we should no longer be discussing whether campaigns are effective but rather how much they achieve by average size effect. She notes the baseline average of a 5% change effect of campaigns, and highlights health topics that score the highest include seatbelt use, dental care and adult alcohol reduction with the lowest size effect in youth alcohol and drug campaigns.

The media have not just been utilised for behavioural change and they prove a versatile tool in the achievement of health promotion aims. Health practitioners have used media to engage in *agenda setting, coalition building*, challenging health damaging behaviour, promoting policy change, increasing acceptability and challenging stigma alongside other strategies to achieve health-related gains. This demonstrates the power and versatility of mass media, which is further evolving with advances in IT (see Chapter 5).

Mass media may also be a cost effective use of resources. This is partly due to the wide exposure mass media promise for relatively low levels of cost per population. Hogan et al. (2005) suggest that mass media campaigns may efficiently transmit information about HIV transmission as part of a wider strategy to reduce HIV in developing countries and Wang and Labarthe (2011) note in a review that there is economic evidence in favour of reducing intake of sodium through the mass media. Consider the example of one television advertisement aired in a prime spot on Saturday night which can potentially reach more than 10 million viewers for relatively little cost per head.

Mass media have the ability to reach a large number of people simultaneously across wide geographical regions. However, one of the problematic areas of mass media use centres on exposure which is usually passive and campaigns often compete with commercial and private sectors who use media to create an arena filled with persuasive product marketing and powerful social norms (Wakefield et al., 2010). Take the example of the prime spot television advertisement again, even though the potential viewer audience is huge, viewers may leave the room, ignore messages or switch channels during the advertisement break thus reducing the potential impact.

Early beliefs around mass media use centred around the apparent powerful effect of messages on the receiving audience, often referred to as the 'hypodermic needle' approach. It was prophesised that whole populations would heed mass media health education messages and adapt their behaviour accordingly. Of course if this were the case societies worldwide would be filled by populations who drink alcohol sensibly, do not smoke tobacco, eat reduced-fat diets rich in essential vitamins and minerals and engage in other protective and preventative behaviours. This view neglects the macro-level factors that impact on health such as politics, finance or community resources and the micro-level factors such as individual choice, attitudes and beliefs. Although health practitioners are now more realistic about the outcomes of media use, it still remains attractive due to its wide-reaching, appealing, powerful nature.

Mass media are any type of broadcast, printed or electronic communication medium that is sent to the population at large. For the purpose of this textbook, mass media will be divided into four broad categories: audio-visual broadcast media, audio-visual non-broadcast media, print-based media and electronic media. Figure 4.1 illustrates this division in more detail and provides examples of how these categories are used in health promotion work.

Type of media	Example of media	Ways to use media
Audio-visual broadcast media	Television, radio	News programmes, documentaries, soap-operas, education–entertainment, public service announcements (PSAs), advertisements
Audio-visual non-broadcast media	DVDs, videos, CDs	Self-help packages, *vignettes*, documentaries, short features, cartoons, teaching skills
Print media	Newspapers, magazines, leaflets, pamphlets, booklets, journals, books, flyers, photo-comics, billboards, bus wraps	News items, magazine features, advertisements, stories, reports, cartoons, storyboards, experimental marketing
Electronic media	Internet, mobile phones, computer packages, pod casts, social media	Websites, self-help packages, information packages, SMS (short messaging services), blogs, various social media

Figure 4.1   The four categories of mass media

Audio-visual broadcast media include television and radio. These could be used in the creation of news items, the advertisement of health products, public health service announcements or even in soap-opera and dramas. Audio-visual non-broadcast media refers to media that are not broadcast over a recognised channel. This could include CDs or DVDs, and could be used to give information via a short feature or programme, a short documentary, or in the provision of self-help information. Print-based media (often the most widely used in health promotion) includes newspapers, magazines, leaflets and billboards. Print media can be used for information given via leaflets, coverage of a health topic in a news item, short stories, cartoons or magazine features. Electronic media (discussed in depth in Chapter 5) include the Internet, social media, mobile phones and other electronic media. These could be used to provide information or behavioural support through websites or SMS (text messages) but often require users to actively seek information as they tend to involve more user engagement (e.g. searching for information and reading this information when it is found).

ACTIVITY 4.1
Different media sources

Hanks et al. (2012) found that convenience and taste are strong determinants of food choice. Think about the different types of media sources described in Figure 4.1:

1 How could you promote healthy eating using different mass media sources focusing on convenience and taste of healthier foods?
2 Give examples of the type of media you could use, and what messages you could transmit though these sources.

Green and Tones (2011) consider that there are currently four main areas of debate in health promotion in the use of mass media:

1 Mass media as an unhealthy influence, for example, promoting behaviours that are health damaging (e.g. tobacco, alcohol or violence).
2 The marketing of unhealthy products (e.g. high fat foods).
3 The acceptability of using mass media to achieve health promotion goals (over other methods).
4 The division between 'selling health' versus 'giving choices'.

The first point includes the role of the mass media at large. Mass media can promote health-damaging behaviours, and thus the goal of health promotion in utilising media and general mass media use embody contradictory aims. Point 2 can also be included under this umbrella. Mass media as a whole generally do not print health stories through a concern of the promotion of health and the prevention of ill health, but rather because they are newsworthy and topical. Point 3 is linked to the use of media over other methods such as interpersonal communication, which is reputed to have more of an impact than a mass media campaign but is much more time consuming and costly. Mass media may not be the most effective method of communication in all cases, yet it is often the one that is most used. Point 4 refers to the debates around social marketing and selling health, rather than offering a choice or empowering people to choose. This is still an area of debate, but generally health practitioners have been leaning towards using social marketing principles in health communication to increase effectiveness in recent years (see social marketing section later in this chapter).

COMMON MASS MEDIA USE IN HEALTH PROMOTION

Television

Most mass media rely on large-scale mass media mechanisms such as television. Television is the leading source of media information about health issues (Risi et al., 2004) and can potentially reach the widest audience. In countries like the UK television offers the possibility of reaching lower income groups' who are less inclined to engage in health campaigns through traditional channels such as via health centres. Television has been found to have some positive effects in health promotion; for example, in an examination of mass media use among recent quitters of smoking, television advertisements were identified as the most helpful to those trying to stop smoking (Beiner et al., 2006). Supporting this Vallone et al. (2011) found that smokers' awareness of television quit smoking advertisements increased chances of quitting by 24% compared to those who were unaware.

Radio

Radio has been used to promote health through advertisements, education–entertainment (or edutainment) programmes and in public service announcements (PSAs). One of the advantages of radio is the different formats and stations that appeal to a range of listeners. The use of edutainment is showing rising popularity in low income countries in particular, and refers to the use of educational messages integrated into a fictional context. Creel et al. (2011) found that HIV-related stigma, (particularly fear of casual contact) was reduced through the 'Malawi radio diaries', which featured people with HIV telling stories about their everyday lives. In the UK, programmes such as *The Archers* (a radio soap-opera) have created a number of storylines around health issues such as breast cancer (TeHIP, 2005), indicating a move towards the use of entertainment–education principles. One alternative way of using the radio is through PSAs. These are free ways to utilise media and are not as commonly used in the UK as in other countries (such as the US). This may represent a missed opportunity in the UK as radio tends to be reasonably cost effective as advertisements remain relatively inexpensive. There has been some reported success of radio. For example, Hall et al. (2010) suggest that radio stations are ideal media to reach African American audiences and emphasise its unique nature in promoting public health with this group for example; literacy is less important, and radio can provide an interactive forum such as the provision of conversational platforms. Radio can attract specific audience groups. Consider the differences for example in listeners to stations that play rock music, country music, popular music, grunge music, bangra music or gospel music. Potentially messages could be targeted to different audiences who may share some common characteristics.

Print-based media

Historically posters were one of the main media to disseminate health messages. Evaluations on their effectiveness are mixed, showing posters have increased changes in knowledge and attitudes but usually have limited impact on behaviours by themselves (i.e. without supporting campaign materials) (Gorsky et al., 2010). Leaflets have shown some consistent results in raising health awareness and other print-based media have been found to demonstrate positive outcomes. Evidence is growing to support pictorial health warnings on tobacco packets which have been found to improve knowledge and quit-related behaviours (Hoek et al., 2010). O'Hegarty et al. (2006) found that warning labels are used to promote interest in quitting, and also propose that text plus graphic warning labels (such as those in Canada) may be more effective than text only. Overall print media demonstrate more effectiveness when combined with other methods and good design principles (see Corcoran, 2011).

Multi-media

Research suggests that the use of a selection of mass media channels is more likely to result in an effective campaign (Peterson et al., 2005; Wakefield et al., 2010). This could include a wide range of media. For example in the LoveLife campaign in South Africa to reduce HIV transmission and change risky sexual practice mass media included television and radio messages, billboards and a free monthly magazine supported by school and community events and programmes (Taylor et al., 2010). The UK Change4Life (DH, 2009a) also makes use of a wide range of media sources including television and radio advertisements, posters, leaflets, a website and various paper-based resources such as family food diaries and stickers. A number of authors suggest multi-media methods are the most effective in achieving campaign aims. For example characteristics of effective campaigns aimed at increasing antibiotic use in outpatient departments illustrate that multi-media use is the most commonly used strategy (e.g. using posters, leaflets, television and radio) and support the finding that multi-faceted campaigns are the most effective (Huttner et al., 2010). See also Case Study 4.1.

Case Study 4.1

Tales of the Road

The UK Department for Transport (DfT, 2012b) uses multi-media for the road safety campaign for children 'Tales of the Road' (see Figure 4.2). This campaign is aimed at 6- to 11-year-olds based on research that children in this age range need to understand the reasons for always practising good road safety behaviour. Animated characters are chosen as they are vulnerable to the consequences of not following good road use. The key message is 'you need to use good road safety behaviour or you could come to real harm'. A variety of resources are available including a toolkit for classroom settings.

More information is available at www.talesoftheroad.direct.gov.uk.

It is also important to remember that the difference for some of the larger multi-media campaigns is their heavy resource base (e.g. funding, facilities, resources), something small-scale campaigns may not have. More frequently the focus has been on 'multi-component' interventions which include other methods (e.g. community events) alongside media to increase effectiveness. For example Knai et al. (2006) and Van Cauwenberghe et al. (2010) suggest multi-component interventions are the most successful in increasing fruit and vegetable intake in children. Case Study 4.2 and Activity 4.2 consider evidence in multi-component mass media interventions in more detail.

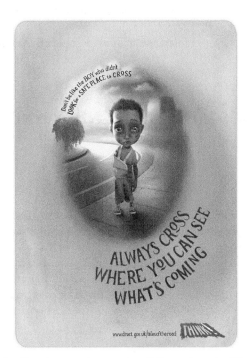

Figure 4.2 Tales of the Road campaign poster, © Department of Transport 2012

Mass media, tobacco use and young people

- Bates et al. (2003) propose that a national tobacco campaign should include public communication programmes which use mass media, and that these should be used to de-normalise and create an emotional response in smokers. They recommend giving a low priority to school-based initiatives, youth access initiatives (restricting access to under-16s, for example) and youth 'counter-marketing' strategies (which can strengthen appeal to cigarettes).
- Farrelly et al. (2003) consider that anti-tobacco advertising campaigns have been demonstrated to have the potential to decrease tobacco use among young people, although these campaigns demonstrate more success when combined with school or community programmes. This finding is fairly consistent for campaigns at a larger level.
- Sowden and Arblaster (2006) conclude that the evidence is not strong for mass media deterring young people from starting smoking.

ACTIVITY 4.2
Mass media and tobacco

Based on the evidence in Case Study 4.2:

1 How do you think mass media should be used (if at all) to prevent tobacco use in young people?
2 What methods could you combine with (or use instead of) mass media?

WHAT THE MASS MEDIA CAN AND CANNOT DELIVER

The mass media can . . .

- *Achieve wide coverage:* One of the main reasons why media are so popular are their promise of exposure to a wider audience and potential large-scale coverage at a reasonably low cost.
- *Impact on behaviours receptive to change:* Wakefield et al. (2010) suggests that behaviour that is episodic such as screening, or one-off rather than habitual, e.g. physical activity, is more likely to change through mass media. In addition it is easier to change a behaviour already being performed or maintain a healthy

behaviour that is already being performed (e.g. choosing a higher factor sun screen and applying it more frequently).

- *Convey simple information:* Mass media can convey simple information and change behaviour if the wider environment supports behaviour change. For example, a message that encourages physical activity five times a week could change the behaviour of someone who currently exercises three times a week who has a subscription to a local gym, and who would then have two extra sessions for no extra fee.
- *Increase knowledge:* Mass media can increase knowledge; for example Barbor et al. (2003) found that mass media campaigns around alcohol and drugs have been found to increase knowledge.
- *Put health on the public agenda:* Mass media can help raise health interest in the general public; for example, celebrities such as Kylie Minogue and Jade Goody who have publicly battled with breast cancer and cervical cancer respectively have been linked to the increased rates of screening for both cancers during these media stories (Holmes, 2010). Media advocacy (discussed later in this chapter) and utilising the media for free via newspapers or magazines can also increase public awareness of health issues.

Hands only CPR

'Hard and fast' and 'Hands only CPR' are the campaign messages for the British Heart Foundation (BHF, 2012) to promote knowledge and increase the skills of those able to perform CPR (cardiopulmonary resuscitation). They use a UK actor and ex-footballer in a short video (Vinnie Jones) to try and increase knowledge of CPR techniques. The campaign message from Vinnie Jones is 'let me teach you a lesson you'll never forget'. The campaign includes a television advertisement and a website with a blog, pocket CPR app, an Ask Vinnie questions section, as well as music, T-shirts and other campaign materials.

For more information go to www.bhf.org.uk.

Case Study 4.3

Case Study 4.3 is an example of what mass media can do. It is still hotly debated just how much the mass media can achieve. Research suggests that there are some areas where mass media are not an appropriate method, as explained below.

The mass media cannot ...

- *Change structural, political or economic factors:* Mass media remain powerless to change factors that may be the main underlying cause of morbidity and mortality. For example in Kenya mass media were positively associated not only with spousal communication of HIV prevention but also with household wealth and status (Chiao et al., 2011). While a practitioner can work to increase exposure to mass media, changing household wealth and status will be a much harder task. Wakefield et al. (2010) also note that access to key services and products and policies that support change are crucial to success in designing mass media campaigns and represent a complementary strategy in campaign design. On a more positive note mass media can assist in changing wider societal structures through mechanisms such as coalition building or advocacy.

- *Change behaviour without facilitating factors:* If facilitating factors are evident change is more likely. For example mass media campaigns can be used to change smoking-related cognitions or prompt quitting behaviours when combined with other methods of tobacco control (Vallone et al., 2011) such as social or political contexts that influence choices. Media advocacy may be a potential strategy that can impact on healthy choices (see later discussion in this chapter).

- *Provide face-to-face support:* One of the features of mass media is that they reach a mass audience and thereby do not communicate with populations on an interpersonal level. Including helpline numbers, SMS (text messaging) services, social media or websites as part of media campaigns can increase the level of individual support (see Chapter 5).

- *Teach a skill (or skills):* The very nature of media (one message to all) mitigates against teaching a skill especially complex ones such as cooking skills, and thus other communication methods need to be used to facilitate acquirement of a skill. Romer at al. (2009) note that face-to-face interventions allow for active participation, i.e. skills training which mass media cannot provide. A multi-component intervention may be necessary for skill acquisition.

- *Convey complex information:* Mass media cannot convey complex information, and simple messages remain the best media messages (see Case Study 4.4). Mazor et al. (2010) examined comprehension of spoken information aired on television and the Internet in cancer prevention and screening and found that while the main messages were generally comprehended, problems included over-generalisation, loss of detail and confusion or misunderstanding of the messages. Complex information is better presented in formats that allow for audience control, i.e. a booklet.

- *Change strong attitudes or beliefs:* Attitudes and beliefs are often deeply ingrained (see Chapter 2), and mass media alone will find it hard to change these. Bradbury (2009) notes that despite evidence (from the NHS, numerous studies and a systematic review of the evidence) to suggest that the MMR vaccine is safe, some parents and medical professionals are still convinced that the vaccine is linked to Cohn's disease or autism and vaccination rates in some areas have decreased dramatically. To address these attitudes and beliefs campaigns may need a variety of strategic communication methods.

To counter-balance these advantages and disadvantages, a number of strategies may be utilised. First, a combination of methods should be employed. Mass media should be used in conjunction with other programmes that contain interpersonal interactions, such as community-based programmes, and should acknowledge possible limitations. Mass media have a key role to play in health, but only when combined with an integrated approach that utilises other agencies, resources or methods. For example, there is evidence to suggest that television advertisements (designed to highlight smoking-related illness in two cigarette pictorial warning topics) and health warnings on cigarette packets (designed by tobacco manufacturers) complement each other and increase motivation to quit (Brennan et al., 2011). In addition multi-agency approaches that are targeted, well timed and support facilitation of behaviour change where possible are needed.

Second, the planned campaign needs to have realistic expectations about what it can achieve in line with the programme aims. If a programme wants to teach a skill, for example, physical activity chair exercises for older people, mass media might not be appropriate. However, if a programme wanted to raise awareness of risks of skin cancer through basic sun safety, mass media could be the appropriate choice.

ACTIVITY 4.3
Suitability of methods for mass media

1 Decide which of the activities below could be achieved through the mass media.
2 For those that are unsuitable for mass media, which methods would you suggest instead?

   i   Raising awareness of risk factors in CHD (coronary heart disease) in males above 40.
   ii The opening of a national new 'stop smoking' helpline.
   iii Increasing the number of young women who are screened for cervical cancer.
   iv Enabling young children to have the skills to cross the road safely.
   v   Changing negative attitudes to schizophrenia.

CREATING A HEALTH CAMPAIGN USING MASS MEDIA

It has been suggested that there are conditions that can help to facilitate a successful campaign. A range of authors advocate a solid theoretical basis to mass media campaigns (Brinn et al., 2010; Dale and Hanbury, 2010; Sowden and Arblaster, 2006). General consensus also highlights the importance of formative research in the design of campaign messages (Brinn et al., 2010; Noar, 2006). Additional variables such as reasonable intensity, audience segmentation and targeting and evaluation are also postulated as successful elements of a mass media campaign. Understanding of the determinants of behaviour targeted in a campaign could lead to the desired health behaviour being performed (Randolf and Viswanath, 2004). As behaviour is influenced by factors defined in theories, it is helpful to choose a theory that fits the aim and objectives of the campaign (see Chapter 1), alongside wider socially, psychologically and culturally appropriate messages (see Chapter 2).

Campaigns utilising mass media that are targeted to a certain group of the population can have a modest impact and those designed with a particular audience in mind will be the most effective (Wilson, 2007). Effectively researched, well-planned and developed campaigns have higher success and are more likely to last longer (Sowden and Arblaster, 2006) and campaigns are often criticised for their lack of rigorous design which may lead to only reporting weak effects (Romer et al., 2009). Noar (2006) proposes that the more a campaign designer adheres to the principles behind an effective campaign design, the more success can be seen in the uses of mass media in health campaigns. There is increasing evidence that media in campaigns can be effective, providing that programmes adhere to the principles of the campaign design (Noar, 2006).

1	**Conduct formative research (pre-target group)** Examine evidence base Consider rationale for campaign
2	**Use theory** Framework and foundation to the campaign
3	**Segment audience** Identify target group demographics including social and psychological factors, social marketing strategies
4	**Message design** Aims/objectives of campaign targeted to segment audience Choose novel, creative methods
5	**Use chosen/appropriate channels from target group** Medium, exposure, duration
6	**Transmit message** Send the message via the correct channels
7	**Conduct evaluation; process, impact and outcome** Check implementation, exposure, recall and effectiveness Match to campaign objectives

Figure 4.3   Designer success, based on Noar's (2006) principles for effective design of mass media campaigns

Figure 4.3 illustrates the basic campaign design steps that should be included in a mass media campaign. Although this is a simplified version of processes that a health practitioner would undertake, it provides a checklist of key stages in campaign design. First, it is suggested that pre-research is conducted to determine the target group and the rationale for the campaign. Locating existing literature and examination of the evidence base is also important. Second, the use of theory should be employed. The theoretical models as described in Chapter 1 can be adapted and applied to programme design. The third stage is audience segmentation. This includes identifying the target group's *demographics*, influential social and psychological factors, and may also include social marketing principles. The fourth stage is designing the message. This includes formulating the aims and objectives of the campaign, and then designing and testing a message for the target audience. The fifth stage is the selection of appropriate mass media channels, and how the information will be transmitted through these channels including length, duration and timing. After transmission of the message the last stage includes conducting an evaluation to check the implementation of the message, exposure and recall to enable determination of the success of campaign objectives.

All health campaigns should include an evaluation plan. It is difficult to measure effectiveness (Hill, 2004) and exposure levels are often estimated, although this does not always give a true measure of what has been achieved. Recall and recognition measures would help the designer to see how successful the message was in achieving exposure (Randolf and Viswanath, 2004). See Chapter 7 for more information on evaluating health promotion work.

TARGET GROUPS AND MESSAGE DESIGN

Peterson et al. (2005) suggest clear identification of the target group to enable design of phrases that will motivate them: 'for a target group to be aware of a campaign . . . it must be memorable' (Peterson et al., 2005: 438), therefore choosing and creating an appropriate message is essential. Message pre-testing is vital to counteract any identified negative impacts or unplanned effects of a message. Pre-testing should include checking to see if the message is salient, understood and memorable (Russell et al., 2005), alongside the more traditional message testing of reception, comprehension and response to the message. See Figure 4.4 for guidelines for re-writing or designing written materials.

Simple messages in current media

- 'Hard and fast' – for hands only CPR (British Heart Foundation 2012)
- 'Think bike: Think biker' – Department for Transport road safety campaign for motor-bikes (DfT 2012c)
- 'Talk to Frank' – UK government campaign for drug knowledge and awareness (ongoing) (Talk to Frank 2012).
- 'Change4Life' – UK Department of Health healthy lifestyles campaign (DH 2009a ongoing)
- 'Know what you're getting into' Part of London Metropolitan Police Cab Wise campaign (Metropolitan Police 2006 ongoing) to discourage illegal minicab use.

Case Study 4.4

1	**Conduct a readability test using members of the target group** Can your target group understand all the words and their meanings? Is the material logical? Consistent? Coherent?
2	**Re-write complex information including unusual or difficult words, and remove any 'jargon'** Which parts are complicated or need further explanation? Are the main message(s) simple? Would headings help to segment information?
3	**Use 'our'/ 'we' to maintain a collaborative voice, rather than 'you'** Does the material seek to make people feel included in the text? Are all the materials in the same style and tense?
4	**Simplify complex tables and diagrams** Are the tables/diagrams necessary? Are they easy to understand from a lay perspective?
5	**Use a glossary of difficult terms** Are there complex words which may need further explanation?
6	**Re-conduct a readability test and pilot on the target group** Do the target audience fully comprehend the revised material?

Figure 4.4   Brief guidelines for re-writing, or designing written material

The development of a message, themes and appropriate images needs to be done in close conjunction with the target group (Sowden and Arblaster, 2006). An example is the work by the Portman Group, who recommend when targeting messages at young women that the focus should be on what excessive drinking could lead to. These include walking home alone, accepting lifts from people they don't know, as well as unsafe sex and how female appearance can be affected by alcohol (DH, 2004). Bates et al. (2003) suggest choosing propositions, for example 'I worry that if I do not stop smoking I will not see my children grow up', or 'I worry that smoking will harm the health of my baby'. For these propositions themes, images and messages can be developed in close conjunction with the target group. See Case Study 4.5.

Thematic words

Peterson et al. (2005) used thematic words to develop messages to promote exercise in 18- to 30-year-olds. They asked the target group to write down a two or three word phrase that came to mind in the promotion of exercise. Final chosen words included 'fun' and 'my appearance'. Results suggested that the final theme and design should include a range of fun activities shown to promote health, alongside highlighting that physical activity will help you to 'look good' in a 'party setting' focus.

Case Study 4.5

ACTIVITY 4.4
A sensible drinking campaign message

Using the Case Study 4.5, try to develop a campaign message for encouraging sensible drinking in 18- to 25-year-olds:

1   List as many key words that you can think of for 'sensible drinking' and '18–25', along with motivations to 'drink sensibly'.
2   Choose two or three of these words to use as your main campaign theme words.
3   Try to formulate these into a phrase or slogan that your campaign could use.

Once a message has been formulated, exposure to the message needs to be substantial for there to be any effect (Farrelly et al., 2003). Both repetition of the message alongside refreshment of messages (e.g. different images or slogans) can also help exposure and impact. Hoek et al. (2010) suggest in reference to effective pictorial health warnings on tobacco packets that frequent image development and refreshment is important alongside recognising concerns held by different smoker sub-groups. This suggests keeping messages 'fresh' may retain interest in the campaign for longer.

SOCIAL MARKETING

Social marketing applied to health is 'the systematic application of marketing concepts and techniques to achieve specific behaviour goals relevant to improving health and reducing health inequalities' (NSMC, 2011). It uses commercial marketing strategies that involve a voluntary behaviour change. Social marketing uses a systematic framework that integrates key strategies that can be used to help inform the planning, design and development of communication interventions. In recent years it has been integrated into health campaigns more rigorously as practitioners realise how the use of models developed in other sectors could translate into health practice. Recent research suggests potential for integration into a wide range of health topics including mental health stigma and HIV testing (see Thackeray et al., 2011).

Social marketing is more than just mass communication. It takes into account a wide spectrum of influences, including economics, legal measures and policy (Green and Tones, 2011). It has been argued for example that condom social marketing has increased condom supplies, broadened commercial markets for condoms and introduced marketing innovations in developing countries (Knerr, 2011). An example from Pakistan (Agha and Beaudoin, 2012) notes that awareness of a social marketing campaign for a brand of condoms increase belief in effectiveness, and the use of, condoms. This suggests the potential of social marketing to not only impact on health behaviours, but societal and economic factors. Chapter 9 has some additional examples of social marketing campaigns that are not covered in this chapter.

Social marketing frameworks have proved to be particularly adaptable, and marketing principles can be used in a variety of ways in health campaigns. The advantages of social marketing include 'features' applicable to each stage of the campaign design, for example, clear target group identification. Because social marketing follows a clear framework it becomes easier to identify constraints and enabling factors to performing behaviours. There is growing evidence to suggest that social marketing can improve the impact and effectiveness of campaigns (NSMC, 2011).

Some health practitioners have taken social marketing concepts fully on board and have integrated social marketing into large-scale health promotion campaigns. For example, in the US, the VERB campaign launched in 2002 aimed to promote the benefits of physical activity, self-efficacy and social influences in a theory-based campaign targeted at 'tweens' (children aged 9–13). This means the campaign used messages such as it's social, cool and fun, rather than traditional messages emphasising the benefits, to promote physical activity through a variety of methods such as commercial marketing techniques, i.e. paid television advertising and advertising in magazines alongside school and community-based activities (Huhman et al., 2010).

The success of social marketing is based around a variety of 'features'. These include the segmentation of audiences, consumer research, competition, exchange theory, monitoring and the marketing mix (or the four Ps) and interactions between interpersonal media and the mass media (Grier and Bryant, 2005). The consensus tends to be that using the whole social marketing process, rather than taking one element (e.g. the four Ps) will result in a more effective campaign.

Audience segmentation

Social marketing borrows techniques from commercial marketing including identifying target groups and their 'consumer orientation'. The American Dietetic Association for example segments adults into three groups based on opinion polls of people's nutritional beliefs and behaviours. These are 'I'm already doing it', 'I know I should but . . .' and 'don't bother me' (Wilson, 2007). The final group being the hardest to change. Each group is thoroughly researched and messages are pre-tested on this group. Social marketing splits populations into sub-groups based on psychological and social characteristics and behaviours. In health promotion the same process can be applied to practice in a target group (see Chapter 2).

ACTIVITY 4.5
Audience segmentation

In sexual health interventions there are a variety of groups that could be targeted for sexual health promotion messages. Using an audience segmentation strategy, these groups would be split into sub-groups.

For example, one group that might benefit from an HIV prevention message could be 11- to 15-year-old secondary school children. They could be divided into male and female, then sexually active and non-sexually active. In the sexually active group they could further be split into contraceptive users and non-contraceptive users and so on.

Using the example of a campaign that aims to encourage regular diabetes checks in those that are diabetic:

1   Identify the groups that could be targeted for this message.
2   Choose one of these groups and identify what characteristics (e.g. male/female) or behaviours (e.g. regular management/non-management) allow 'segmentation' into further sub-groups. Think about the social/psychological factors from Chapter 2.

Consumer research

The concept is that what the consumer wants and needs should form the basis of a social marketing strategy. This means researching the target group's needs, preferences, opinions, beliefs and other areas that impact on behaviour. The move to include evidence-based practice in health promotion is particularly useful for substantiating these findings.

Competition

Social marketing will have thoroughly researched the competition and what product or service they are offering. In health promotion this could include identifying unhealthy behaviours that compete with healthy ones, as well as examining other health messages that are being marketed.

Exchange theory

It is postulated that consumers buying a product will weigh up the pros/cons or benefits/costs. The product bought will more likely be the one with the greatest benefit at the least cost. These costs are not just financial, but can also include time, pleasure, habit, enjoyment and others. In application to health promotion, the benefits of the behaviour need to be highlighted alongside recognition of the costs. For example, stopping smoking could be something that a person enjoys and uses as stress relief (the benefits of smoking) versus advantageous reasons for stopping, including more money or a decrease in respiratory problems (the costs of smoking).

Monitoring

Social marketing uses evaluation from the start of the planning process to the end. In health promotion, evaluation is fundamental to check that programmes are achieving their objectives, and all health promotion programmes should include process, impact and outcome evaluation (see Chapter 8).

The four Ps

In addition to audience segmentation, exchange theories and competition, social marketing also borrows a marketing mix known as the four (or five) Ps. These Ps are *Product, Price, Place, Promotion,* and sometimes a fifth additional variable *Positioning.* They form the central core of any social marketing plan, and their attractiveness lies in their ease of application to health promotion work:

- *Product:* The characteristics of the product (or behaviour), i.e. attractiveness.
- *Price:* The costs, value and importance of performing a behaviour (actual and imagined), including social, economic, psychological costs.
- *Place:* Where the product (or behaviour) is available.
- *Promotion:* Where the product is sold, including publicity, message design and distribution.
- *Positioning:* Framing issues so that the target group remembers them.

This marketing mix could be applied to health behaviour and campaign design (see Case Study 4.6).

ACTIVITY 4.6
The four Ps

Following the four Ps framework described above, apply it to the following activity:
A health promotion campaign to increase uptake of breastfeeding in first time mothers (the Product) in a small community.

1 Identify what Price, Place, Promotion and Positioning you could use to promote breastfeeding in this group.

The four Ps

In the US a three-month social marketing campaign was undertaken to raise awareness among parents and reduce barriers to accessing the vaccine for routine immunisation against human papillomavirus (HPV). The campaign targeted mothers of girls aged 11–12. The four Ps that were used in the campaign were:

- *Product:* The recommended vaccine against HPV.
- *Price:* Cost, perception of safety and efficacy, access.
- *Place:* Doctor's offices and retail outlets.
- *Promotion:* posters, brochures, website, news releases and doctors' recommendations.
  (Cates et al., 2011)

CRITICISMS OF SOCIAL MARKETING

Although promising for health promotion work, social marketing is not without its critics. Social marketing is challenged with both trying to change behaviour for benefits that are not always guaranteed (e.g. reducing the risks of CHD) and they may not become apparent for a long period of time (Plant et al., 2010). The focus of social marketing on individuals rather than the broader determinants of health have come under some criticism too (see Grier and Bryant, 2005). Accusations of providing simple problems which act as a 'quick fix' to much larger issues (Gagnon et al., 2010) surround the use of social marketing alongside the absence of environmental or political factors in campaigns. The most common criticism is that social marketing is 'manipulative' as it persuades people to be healthy in the same way that consumers are persuaded to buy products. This borrowing of what Hill (2004) refers to as 'manipulative techniques' has led to questions around ethical issues of social marketing.

In defence of social marketing, however, the 'consumer research' aspect proposes that the consumer (or audience) defines their own wants and needs when 'buying' a product. In health, therefore, involving the target group in all the pre-planning processes enables the target group to 'buy' the healthy product that they want. In addition, as social marketing is used more frequently, voluntary choice rather than coerced behaviour change, is emphasised. Involvement in social marketing may also encourage health practitioners to look towards environmental or societal impacts.

Grier and Bryant (2005) note social marketing's tendency to be expensive and inappropriate for small-scale projects, however a social marketing study targeting 7000 heroin users in the US suggests differently. The study notes that the costs of ethnographic mapping of injection drug use and producing and distributing posters and newsletters only comes to a fraction of the lifetime cost of treating a single HIV infection (see Gibson et al., 2010). The principles applied in a social marketing framework reflect the more traditional planning frameworks in health promotion.

This suggests a productive move to ally theoretical principles closely with practice, which is a positive step for health practitioners and their health promotion work.

BRANDING HEALTH

One practice that is closely linked to social marketing is branding health campaigns. Research suggests that branding a campaign can increase the impact of a campaign (Vallone et al., 2011). Evidence from commercial marketing indicates that the more an audience likes an advertisement, the more they like the brand marketed in the message (Cho and Choi, 2010). In addition, key recognition of people, places or colours can influence choices, for example media cartoon characters can influence children's food choices (Kotler et al., 2012). Plant et. al. (2010) stipulate that branding is more than just a name or a logo, but an emotional response that a product can evoke and acts as a 'mental shorthand' (p. 24) meaning that information about a product can be easily recalled. A strong brand can increase campaign impact especially when the target group endorses the product or behaviour. In health the emphasis is often on the adoption of a new behaviour over an old one (rather than choosing to buy one product over another).

Priming may also be a useful part of branding, for example if a target audience can recognise a brand before the campaign starts the impact may be greater. This is a strategy that many non-health products employ before the release of products. For example, a variety of products are promoted through fast-food giveaways, or magazine tokens before they are actually released to buy. Ma et al. (2011) suggest priming in relation to a public health campaign on cardiovascular risks can increase awareness and knowledge and may promote behaviour change. In a health promotion context in the US the New York City Department of Health and Mental Hygiene created the 'NYC condom', unique to New York City, which reported high rates of use particularly in high-risk persons (see Burke et al., 2011 for further details) suggesting a possible affinity to the product and the associations connected with NYC.

UTILISING THE MEDIA FOR FREE

Health in the news and newspapers

Recent research suggests that the concept of health is evolving to include issues that threaten health security, for example swine flu (H1N1) that crosses geographical boundaries. This creates a bias in the reporting of health stories and may neglect important and key issues. In addition, as the focus on news is to 'sell a story' the key facts may be missing or misleading an audience. For example McCartney (2011) notes the problems between reporting relative risk and excluding absolute risk in scientific papers and press releases which may give inaccurate information to the general public (in this case the polypill, which when absolute risk is considered does not 'half' heart disease or stroke as claimed in the news). An imbalance in topics that are reported is also problematic, or the style in which they are reported, leading to health scares. Topics of interest often tend to be those that impact on relatively few, but have a sensational interest such H1N1, or that herald a scientific breakthrough. As newspapers often reflect public attitudes and interest, this imbalance should be of interest to the health practitioner. If current media interest is not focused towards health promotion, the general population, policy-makers and governments will also rate cure more highly that prevention.

However, newspapers may be one way to place health issues on the public agenda. There is evidence that some media coverage impacts on behaviour. Health scares can generate an increase in health seeking behaviour, and reports on copy-cat behaviour such as suicide are closely linked to the media portrayal of suicide (see Williams, 2011). Policy and government priorities can take cues from the media agenda (Harrabin et al., 2003). Oronje et al. (2011) suggest that in Sub-Saharan Africa the media have a clear potential to promote good sexual and reproductive health outcomes but often fail to prioritise sexual and reproductive health and rights issues or report them in an accurate way. They suggest providing training or competitive grants for outstanding reporting in this area, building capacity of journalists to report in this area and of health researchers to communicate research through the media alongside establishing and maintaining relationships between researchers and journalists.

Health practitioners should take an active approach to media use in health promotion and strive to develop this, for example, including stories in the media that appeal to audiences from human interest angles. Smaller communities will have more opportunities to influence news as the content is usually a reflection of what is happening in that community (Martinson and Hindman, 2005). Health education or health agenda raising in newspapers also have low resource implications.

Media advocacy

Media advocacy is the 'strategic use of mass media for advancing social or public policy initiatives' (MacDonald, 1998: 116). Media advocacy can attempt to change and influence programmes, policies or agendas that can be damaging to health. It has been suggested that print media and *health advocacy* play a strong role in the adoption of policies and laws (Ashbridge, 2006), probably through drawing attention to a particular issue that encourages a response from the policy-maker. Media advocacy may be one way of utilising media to raise public awareness of or influence public policy on a group or community-advocated action. Freudenberg et al. (2009) give examples of areas such as alcohol, food and drink, firearms and pharmaceuticals where news media can play a huge role in framing issues, raising awareness and mobilising groups to promote healthy societies.

On the negative side, there are some organisations and groups in society that promote disease rather than health, or as Freudenberg notes, 'organizational practices or policies that encourage unhealthy behaviours, lifestyles or environments' (2005: 299). For example it can be difficult to quit smoking in the face of widespread tobacco advertising (Khowaja et al., 2010). Another example is the continued use by the fashion and advertising industry of very thin models despite evidence to suggest the general population would prefer greater body size diversity (see, for example, Diedrichs et al., 2011). These 'disease promoting' behaviours can include a variety of factors embodied by organisations who seek to exert power, authority or jurisdiction. They can use media to advertise (unhealthy) products alongside more subtle routes of power, for example by giving funding to a charity, lobbying current governmental departments to support their cause or donating money to fund research. All of these actions have the goal of enabling promotion of their products, thus increasing profits and power. These groups need not be multinational private companies, for example during the partial smoking ban in Greece in 2009, Andreou et al. (2010) argue that newspapers played a negative role in promoting smoking policy change and were pessimistic about law enforcement and Kemp et al. (2011) note the conflicting messages in the media of sun safety which can hamper health promotion efforts.

ACTIVITY 4.7
Media advocacy

1 Make a list of current national organisations or groups who promote products that could be classed as health damaging.
2 Choose one of these, and say how using the media advocacy techniques described above could influence a change to these health-damaging behaviours.

Challenging large organisations can be difficult. Action can include advocating change or influencing organisational practices or policies. This might be through legislative action on the part of the health practitioner or through influencing policy such as restricting the use of advertising. It could also be through responding to news or creating new news items around these health-damaging practices. Media advocacy can include challenging the media themselves, for example in Stop the Sores, a social marketing campaign whose aim was to increase syphilis testing, knowledge and awareness, the commercial media were used for free publicity. The campaign utilised media advocacy when several local television stations refused to air a television advertisement which had already been shown extensively on other television channels. The subsequent press conferences and newspaper articles generated free publicity and a huge increase in website traffic (Plant et al., 2010) proving bad press may also be good press.

Media advocacy has been challenged by some practitioners who argue that there is little evidence to show these companies are damaging the health of others, and that health promotion should look at individual behaviours rather than the wider sphere of health. Others propose it may jeopardise public relations, funding or the neutral role of the health educator (Freudenberg, 2005). Given the fundamental definition of health promotion that includes wider determinants of health, media advocacy is something that should hold more popularity with practitioners. The role played by multinational organisations in society may require responses that differ from the more traditional role of the health educator.

USING INCENTIVES: FEAR APPEALS AND POSITIVE APPEALS

Health promotion has traditionally transmitted messages where audiences usually have to stop doing something, particularly things that are 'comfortable habits . . . and . . . pleasurable experiences' (Monahan, 1995: 81). Usually messages are designed in health to promote fear or present facts in a rational way, which is contradictory to commercial advertising, which rarely uses rational fear-provoking messages but adopts a more positive focus (Monahan, 1995). While health messages encourage people to stop smoking or drink sensibly, among other things, commercial marketing is doing the opposite. Commercial marketing encourages these opposing behaviours through entertaining and engaging audiences to utilise or purchase a product or undertake a behaviour by making the product as attractive as possible.

Fear appeals

A fear appeal is 'threatening the audience with harmful outcomes from initiating or continuing an unhealthy practice' (Atkin, 2001: 61), usually through a message that emphasises possible physical harm or social consequences of failing to comply with the recommended message (Hale and Dillard, 1995). For example, if you drink and drive you may be involved in a serious accident, or if you smoke tobacco you are more likely to die a premature death. Some research suggests their effectiveness. Zaidi et al. (2011) suggest that graphic pictorial multi-media health warnings that focus on functional distortions, for example a picture of an oral cavity or a patient on a ventilator, were more likely to be perceived as an effective anti-smoking message than those that focused on elements such as the impact of smoking on disposable income.

Atkin (2001) considers that well-designed fear appeals can be quite effective in changing behaviours, although they should also show the audience how to change behaviour. Effective fear appeal messages should include a problem-solution framework (Hale and Dillard, 1995). This could be emphasising the threat and the vulnerability of the target audience to that threat and then providing a solution or recommendations to that problem. Green and Witte (2006) propose that fear arousal messages can work if they are combined with self-efficacy skills that could lead to behaviour change. Rarely, however, do mass media interventions allow for the development of self-efficacy skills. It is important to recognise that not all fear appeals work in all circumstances. Messages that confuse or increase fear may be frequently ignored or prove difficult to recall.

ACTIVITY 4.8
Fear appeals

You are designing a poster campaign for young women to raise awareness of the risks associated with the so-called 'date rape' drug Rohypnol from 'spiked' alcoholic drinks.

1 What risks could you highlight associated with this drug for young women?
2 How would you provide a 'solution' to this problem?

Positive appeals

A positive effect message is one that encourages positive feeling, which could in turn influence behaviour or cognitive processes (Monahan, 1995). Peterson et al. (2005) recommend the use of positive reinforcement and the avoidance of negative messages. Positive appeals can be used in a number of ways; they may want to change the audience's current perceptions so the audience views the behaviour from a different perception (e.g. turning physical activity from being seen as uncomfortable or tiring to being a way to meet new friends, or something that is fun). Positive appeals could also provide evidence of how performing behaviour will have a positive outcome, for example, a case study which shows how someone going through a behaviour change has a successful outcome. Positive messages are also likely to be more effective when positive attitudes already exist and messages can reinforce the positive aspects of performing or changing a behaviour though positive framing.

CONCLUSION

Fundamentally, in health promotion, health practitioners should no longer be concerned with debates around whether media work or not as mass media are used extensively to achieve health promotion aims. Practitioners need to think about how the elements of media that do work can be used more effectively in conjunction with multi-media and multi-agency working. A combination of techniques such as utilising social marketing strategies alongside media advocacy may be one solution, alongside a more proactive approach to media use. In the fast-developing world of media and IT, health practitioners should be taking a forward-thinking role towards mass media campaign design. Dale and Hanbury (2010) suggest in an exploratory study of healthy eating programmes that there is a mismatch between the health information provided and the audiences' barriers and social influences that prevent them from eating healthily. Mass media use may therefore need to focus on barriers and influences and consider how these can be tackled rather than reliance on providing information that has little impact on the target group.

Furthermore, practitioners should not attempt to re-do what has already been achieved but should look at what already works (particularly those programmes that are based on theory) and use this in future work. Only when health practitioners ensure that their health messages are as effective, well planned and well designed as the competition can they achieve their goal.

Summary

- This chapter has analysed the role of mass media in health promotion work, with particular attention to what mass media can and cannot achieve.
- The role of theory, supportive environments and message design has been considered, alongside the uses of social marketing in the mass media.
- Alternative means of mass media use have been explored through media advocacy, branding and utilising the media via newspapers.
- The place of incentives and fear appeals in health promotion programmes has been discussed.

ADDITIONAL READING

A further discussion on media advocacy can be found in Freudenburg N, Bradley SP and Serrano M (2009) Public health campaigns to change industry practices that damage health: An analysis of 12 case studies. *Health Education and Behaviour* 36 (2): 230–249.

Strategies and campaign tools for media use be found in Corcoran N (2011) *Working on Health Communication*. Sage, London.

A practical step-by-step social marketing textbook is Weinreich NK (2011) *Hands-on Social Marketing*. Sage, London.

See also the National Social Marketing Centre website, www.thensmc.com/.

5

INFORMATION TECHNOLOGY

NOVA CORCORAN

Learning outcomes:

- Examine the role of IT applications in health promotion practice.
- Explore the application of IT to health promotion interventions.
- Consider ways to overcome the challenges of IT for health promotion practice.

With increasing global development in information technology (IT) alongside the growing need to tackle challenging health issues, new developments in IT are becoming increasingly pertinent to health promotion. The use of IT in health is appealing and increasingly being used in health care as populations are encouraged to utilise modern technology for health information. Health and illness information is widely available to the general public and health professionals alike through the increasing popularity of applications such as the Internet and mobile devices such as tablets and touchscreen phones. One of the main objectives that IT in health should be striving towards is allowing individuals, groups and communities to gain knowledge and information about health issues that can prevent ill health and promote good health easily. Health practitioners need to be familiar with strategies that utilise IT to empower, encourage and educate the general public in the bid for health protection, health development and health improvement.

THE ROLE OF INFORMATION TECHNOLOGY IN HEALTH

In 2010 Kreps and Neuhauser noted that 'there is a communication revolution brewing in the delivery of health care and the promotion of health fuelled by the growth of powerful new health information technologies' (p. 329). New technology such as mobile phones, social networking sites and interactive media applications such as touchscreen tablets all hold promise and potential to promote health. *IT* generally includes all interactive media as opposed to paper-based media. The Internet and its applications, i.e. social networking sites and websites, computer games, mobile phones, digital television and other forms of interactive technology, fall under this umbrella. IT has recently joined the realms of mass media and in the future is arguably set to usurp traditional media as the new way to communicate in the Western world. The use of IT in health promotion is a growing field despite some gaps in research. Currently there are a variety of IT applications that have shown promise, and success, in health promotion campaigns.

The combination of IT applications that work to improve health has sometimes been referred to collectively as *e-health*. E-health includes telecommunication or computer-assisted IT that plays a role in health. These applications have been hailed as offering 'unprecedented opportunities for improving equity in access to health-enhancing global . . . interventions' (Kirigia et al., 2005: 10). This is an optimistic view that suggests a wealth of opportunities for IT. Eysenbach (2001) proposes e-health as an emerging way of thinking rather than a specific list of technologies with an overarching aim to utilise and improve the application of IT. Either definition suggests that e-health is an electronic application with the potential to enhance health. For the purpose of this textbook this definition will exclude aspects that are linked to financial, administrative or clinical data, for example, electronic patient records, telemedicine or decision support systems as these are less important for campaigns. IT holds a number of benefits and challenges to both the lay person and the health practitioner and has been framed as offering opportunities to promote health as well as facilitation of access to health and education needs (Fors and Moreno, 2002). A clear understanding of what IT is capable of achieving, and what barriers might be in the way of this goal, is necessary for all practitioners with an interest in health.

IT in communication has been used for a variety of health topics to deliver diverse health messages using a range of media. This includes to:

- Relay information.
- Enable informed decision-making.
- Promote healthy behaviours including preventive aspects, for example screening.
- Facilitate behaviour change.
- Promote support, for example peer information exchanges, emotional support or social support.
- Promote self-care, risk reduction or self-help.
- Manage demand for health services.
- Facilitate communication.

ACTIVITY 5.1
How could IT be used to . . . ?

1 List ways in which you think IT could promote behaviour change.
2 What possible methods or tools does IT offer that could help you to create a more interactive health campaign?

One of the distinct advantages of IT is the engagement of the audience. Unlike mass media where the audience is seen as a passive receiver of messages, the very nature of IT requires engagement from the user (see Chapter 4 for in-depth coverage of mass media). This way of accessing information from a health promotion perspective enables the user to be actively engaged in information seeking. IT can provide 'increased learning, information seeking, information processing, and individualised knowledge' (Rice, 2001: 28), all processes which form the basic ethos of empowerment in health promotion.

THE POTENTIAL OF INFORMATION TECHNOLOGY IN HEALTH PROMOTION

The desire to use IT in health has arisen due to a variety of challenges rather than one single reason. Wallace (1998) lists several, including the rising costs of health care, changing demographics (e.g. an ageing population), developments in IT and increasing public pressure to include other forms of health care (e.g. complementary medicine). Other challenges may include changing global networks and new health and disease patterns. New technology use is growing in nearly all aspects of health communication (Suggs, 2006). Now patients who visit their general practitioner can go armed with more health information (Hall and Visser, 2000), and health practitioners are expected to respond accordingly to the newly informed patient.

One of the most hailed advantages of IT over the mass media is the move away from the audience as passive recipients of messages towards becoming an active audience. This means IT is more closely situated to the Thackeray and Neiger (2009) model of communication (see Chapter 1). Mass media traditionally direct predominately a one-way message. Interactive media, however, can involve participation, experimentation, goal development and other audience-centred methods that were previously impossible via mass media (Lieberman, 2001). This shift in information seeking in health can be seen as a move towards the fusion of target group involvement in decision-making processes. Users can choose via interactive IT applications that allow them to be actively supported in a health behaviour change or illness. These can include email, calendars, support groups or disease management (Benigeri and Pluye, 2003), all of which include engagement of the target group.

There are other advantages of IT pertinent to the health promotion field. The interactive nature of communication in IT allows content to be adapted, altered or tailored to individual users. Provision of information without face-to-face contact is seen as a considerable benefit of IT alongside providing information for hard-to-reach groups. This allows populations who are geographically far apart to access the same information worldwide.

Health practitioners are increasingly expected to engage in these e-health applications in their daily work. If this is the case, then health promotion needs to make sure IT is used effectively to reap the benefits. One of the main advantages of IT over those of the traditional print media is the ease of designing feedback mechanisms that promote interaction. However, too often e-health applications are not designed to promote interaction and collaboration. They are often focused more on providing information than on exchanging messages. This is disappointing as interactivity may be the key to promoting health behaviours (Kreps and Neuhauser, 2010). The huge growth of *social media* has a major impact on health communication with sites such as Twitter (www.twitter.com) and Facebook (www.facebook.com) pushing healthy and unhealthy messages in their general arena of online interaction. As the local population becomes more media savvy, health practitioners need to keep their own IT skills up to date and adapt their campaign designs to an evolving audience.

Electronic media are a much used source by large proportions of the population and for some groups the main source of health information. Campaigns by organisations such as the London Metropolitan Police recognise this and some of the campaigns focused on reducing rates for violent crime such as knife and gun offences are centred around IT and social media (see www.stoptheguns.org). Other authors note that target groups may use sources such as the Internet as their main source of information, but this does not always meet their health needs. For example Char et al. (2011) note that young, unmarried rural Indian men identify electronic mass media as their main source of reproductive health information but they lack detailed knowledge of various contraceptives.

It is possible that in order for health communication to fully utilise IT it needs to look towards commercial marketing techniques. For example a premium condom brand to promote sales and condom use employed a range of social networking techniques via a variety of digital platforms. This included a new website, a Facebook page, an e-newsletter, viral marketing, banner ads and weblogs, resulting in increased recognition among the target audience of sexually active young people (see Purdy, 2011). These commercial marketing techniques suggest a website alone is no longer sufficient in competing with other organisations to promote health, and that a variety of techniques that appeal to the target group are necessary to create a more robust and effective campaign.

IT for health promotion has utilised a number of media. The most popular in current research and practice is the Internet. Other IT applications that have been used in health communication campaigns include computer-based interventions, mobile computers, touchscreen kiosks, mobile phones, touchscreen tablets, CD-ROMs and more recently the growth of social media which utilise this new technology to create social networks.

THE INTERNET

The Internet is one of the most widely researched applications of IT in health. There has been growing interest in the use of the Internet to deliver health promotion campaigns and a number of studies show a positive impact. Statistics suggest that around 64% of adults in the UK accessed the Internet in 2005, mostly in a home environment (ONS, 2006). Online health promotion has the advantage of wide reach and ease of tailoring messages that focus on persuasive constructs (Mevissen et al., 2011). Koch-Weser et al. (2010) found in a review of Internet health information seekers that users were more likely to be younger, more educated, have higher incomes and consider it important to get personal medical information electronically.

Health information is growing in availability on the Internet (Benigeri and Pluye, 2003) and as access and usage has grown, health seeking behaviours on the Internet have also increased (Cline and Haynes, 2001). Duffy et al. (2002) propose that the Internet could potentially be used for health improvement to equip people with the information that they need. Gainer et al. (2003) support this proposition, and note the Internet is often perceived as a good educational tool as well as a valuable information source. They also note that seeking information on the Internet has become routine practice for users and practitioners.

The Internet is something that offers the chance of interpersonal contact. Message boards, for example, can give advice and encouragement and can be important for understanding health seeking behaviours (Macias et al., 2005). Topics on message boards can be wide-ranging, and given that location is not problematic, different people worldwide can congregate online to discuss the same anxieties, share information or support one another through health changes, illness or health behaviours. Williams et al. (2010) note for example that Internet applications can transcend geographical boundaries and social isolation and overcome challenges of face-to-face interventions for the topic of HIV in MSM (men who have sex with men).

The Internet also boasts widespread access and interactivity (Cline and Haynes, 2001) as well as having the benefits of being able to be accessed informally or anonymously (Berger et al., 2005). All these aspects could contribute to an increase in the facilitation of healthy behaviours, from searching for information, interacting with others about health issues to improving health. Due to its anonymity, the Internet may also encourage health seeking behaviour for sensitive subjects such as sexual health issues or other concerns where a person may be embarrassed or too anxious to seek face-to-face advice. Other advantages of using the Internet include the range of interactive elements (Suggs, 2006). The use of message boards, quizzes, games, calculators (e.g. alcohol units or body mass index [BMI]) can quickly give a response to the user. Interactive resources allow a virtual or actual two-way interaction, for example, via web cameras. Users can become involved in their own health choices or illness management and interactivity may also allow users to question their own attitudes, behaviours or beliefs around health issues. The growth of social networking sites is also important for health promotion campaigns, and may offer a way to reach specific target audiences coupled with interpersonal communication opportunities.

Current research that examines website and Internet-based interventions have found relatively promising results. Physical activity for example has been found to increase through website interventions in the short term (Magnoc et al., 2011; Wadworth and Hallam, 2010) but less promising is the use of IT in long term behaviour change, despite efforts to tailor interventions to theoretical constructs (both using social cognitive theory).

STI risk communication intervention

Case Study 5.1

Williams et al. (2010) aimed to influence risk perceptions and promote the maintenance of condom use and STI (sexually transmitted infection) testing in those recently starting a new homosexual relationship. The setting was a virtual STI public clinic where the visitor (the participant) was guided through the program as if they were in conversation with the virtual consultant. The visitors proceeded through a program using a question and answer format. The consultant asked questions and provided information in text blocks and balloons and participants answered questions by clicking on an answer. Content was focused around three content domains: STI risk perception related to the current relationship, attitude, normative beliefs, self-efficacy and skills towards maintenance of condom use within the current relationship, and STI testing. This allowed for personalised safe sex advice.

ACTIVITY 5.2
Interactive websites

1   What websites can you think of that use interactive resources to promote health?
2   What sort of resources do they use?

Online health promotion and *public health* interventions have increased in recent years. A number of studies have demonstrated the effectiveness of online interventions in a variety of areas. For example a review examining different types of tailored and untailored promotion of fruit and vegetable consumption showed an increase in serving intake (Alexander et al., 2010). Hamel et al. (2010) found that computer and web-based physical activity interventions can promote physical activity particularly in the short term. They also note those interventions based in schools had the biggest impact, suggesting a possible link to supportive settings. They note this style of intervention is capable of reaching large audiences, and those which are theory based and individually tailored offer the most promise. See also Case Study 5.1.

Computer-based interventions have the advantage of being able to include activities such as games, simulations, diary keeping, information finding or goal setting. McDaniel et al. (2005) used an interactive smoking cessation intervention delivered in a clinical setting for inner city women. They found participants reported formulating more behaviour-orientated quit-smoking strategies, suggesting the use of interactivity in goal setting. Burns et al. (2006) suggest that interactive health communication applications have been found to improve knowledge, social support, health behaviours and clinical outcomes. There is also some evidence to suggest the improvement of self-efficacy. In part, some of these outcomes have been linked to the interactive components in these programmes, the mix of visual aids and the opportunity for revisiting information alongside 24-hour access.

Cugelman et al. (2011) suggest that online interventions have the capacity to influence voluntary behaviours and recommend an increase in public health campaigns that mix interpersonal online systems with mass media outreach work. They also note shorter interventions have larger impacts, and greater adherence.

There is a rise in the use of Internet-based tools for self-assessment and testing in relation to health. These are evident on websites such as the Diabetes UK diabetes risk calculator (www.diabetes.org.uk/RiskTest) as well as more complex applications. Zuure et al. (2011) found that Internet-mediated risk-based testing for the hepatitis C virus is an effective way to identify undiagnosed infections in the general population. Participants completed a questionnaire, downloaded a free referral letter for an anonymous hepatitis blood test in a non-clinical setting and accessed the results online one week later. Those who tested positive were referred on for treatment. They also note that those who were infected came predominately from hard-to-reach groups. Barysch et al. (2010) examined an Internet-based interactive education tool for skin cancer prevention (www.skincheck.ch) in Switzerland which was found to increase participation in skin cancer prevention in a middle-aged male population.

Research also suggests the possibility of tailoring health promotion information for culturally specific groups using the Internet. Padilla et al. (2010) found in a focus group for Latinos at risk of heart disease that a website should be:

- Culturally appropriate with images of multigenerational families.
- Colourful, eye-catching, professional.
- Easy to navigate with easy to understand information.
- Interactive with immediate feedback on health.

MOBILE PHONES

Mobile phones are a global phenomenon and in Western countries mobile phone use can be as much as 80% (MORI, 2005). In the UK there are high levels of mobile phone use in most social groups, although older age groups are less likely to use SMS (text messaging) (Atun and Sittampalam, 2006). Mobile phones have the advantage of voice communication alongside SMS, and increasingly access to email, camera facilities and Internet connections. Atun and Sittampalam (2006) herald SMS as having the advantage of being able to be used in different languages, messages can be tailored, stored until read, can be an immediate response and responses can be sent anonymously. In addition there is support in some groups for this mode of intervention, for example Wright et al. (2011) found that young African American men were receptive to the idea of receiving text messages as part of an HIV prevention campaign and Wilkins and Mak (2007) note participants of a chlamydia campaign rated SMS as a good communication strategy.

Figure 5.1 is an example of the Samaritans' (2006) campaign that uses a 24:7 (24 hours, 7 days a week) mobile phone texting service. The charity also uses email as a way of supporting anyone who needs emotional support. They first identified the potential for a text-messaging service in their report that found 94% of 18- to 24-year-olds use mobile phones to send personal messages (Samaritans, 2006), thus providing a rationale for mobile phone support to reach this group.

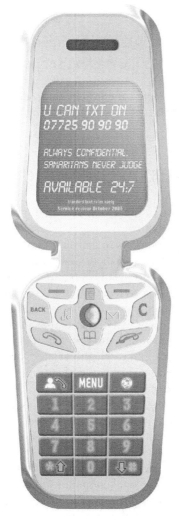

Figure 5.1   The txt Samaritans 4 Emotional Support campaign, © Samaritans 2006

Research has examined the role of SMS applications and health. Atun and Sittampalam (2006) indicate three main advantages: efficiency gains in delivery of health care, benefits to the patient and benefits to public health.

Efficiency gains can include sending appointment reminders to reduce non-attendance at appointments. Da Costa et al. (2010) found that sending appointment reminders as text messages is an effective strategy to reduce non-attendance at outpatient clinics, and Kharbanda et al. (2011) note that HPV vaccine uptake increases through mobile phone reminders. It can benefit patients' compliance to medication or treatment routines, such as oral contraceptive reminders. It has been shown to be effective in increasing adherence to asthma treatment (Strandbygaard et al., 2010). The public health benefits of SMS include communicating health information to the public in emergencies, or the ability to send health promotion advice or support.

ACTIVITY 5.3
SMS messaging services

1   What topics do you think might benefit from the sending of SMS messages?
2   What topics do you think are not as suited to sending via SMS?

ADDITIONAL IT-BASED APPLICATIONS

>> Research suggests an increase in the use of IT-based interventions in health such as *podcasting* and *apps*. Currently the evidence for these areas is scant and studies that have taken place suggest some success in delivery methods (see, for example, Turner-McGrievy and Tate [2011] who use a theory-based podcast for weight loss) but less positive impacts of these interventions in changing behaviours. A touchscreen phone or *tablet* device allows you access to over hundreds of possible healthy lifestyle apps such as calorie counters (of which there are at least 10 different ones; Johnson, 2011) as well as areas such as physical activity related apps including yoga, dance, walking trails, sports trackers and training clubs which require active engagement (e.g. inputting calories) into your phone. Health-related organisations are promoting apps in areas such as surgery recovery and diabetes management. Interestingly, one app store notes that of the free applications that are downloaded after one month below 5% of users are still using the app, and after 3 months it is close to 0% (Spear, 2009). This suggests apps may not be worthwhile in the long term for promoting health, but they may be potentially useful in conjunction with a range of other methods which aim for a long-term change.

Other growth areas in IT include social media such as Twitter, Facebook and interactive blogs for more interpersonal communication (see Corcoran, 2011). Further areas include video games and computer simulation which tend to focus on behaviours such as physical activity or rehabilitation but there may be many more opportunities in health promotion in the future. One of the most useful might be the use of interactive video games. Mejia-Downs et al. (2011) explore the effects of a six-week interactive dance video and note a number of positive health outcomes including some reduction in BMI and respiratory fitness. They also note that active video *gaming* might appeal to groups who are less likely to incorporate physical activity into their lives. It is possible that other virtual simulation arenas such as Second Life (www.secondlife.com) or games consoles that engage the user in physical activity or decision-making processes may also play a future role in health communication interventions.

ADVANTAGES AND DISADVANTAGES OF INFORMATION TECHNOLOGY

In the emerging field of IT in health communication one of the major factors that should be taken into consideration is the identification of what IT is best at achieving. Although fast-growing and hailed as essential to health, IT is not a universal panacea to changing health issues or problems. It is therefore important to consider when communicating health through IT how the communication should be designed, and what the communication is designed for. Health practitioners must take these factors on board and consider how IT can be used to complement or deliver an intervention.

A number of authors have highlighted the advantages and disadvantages of using IT in health promotion. It is important to weigh these up, in the same way as with other traditional methods. As such these barriers have not changed in recent years, and continue to be problematic when creating IT-based health campaigns. Figure 5.2 summarises some of the advantages and disadvantages of IT drawing on the findings of Buller et al. (2001), Lieberman (2001) and Cassell et al. (1998), plus some more recent ideas based on the points raised in this chapter.

Advantages	Disadvantages
• Time saving • Allows tailoring of information to individual needs • Participatory and interactive • Allows user to be proactive and gives choice • Allows feedback to targeted person • Can utilise a variety of different media (e.g. film, audio, pictures) • Allows application of theoretical models into practice • Can be user friendly (e.g. touch screen/voice activation)	• No motivation of targeted person to use programs • Digital divide (i.e. no access to IT or low literacy) • May increase communication inequalities • Competing with other media forms and large companies • Can be costly • Confidentiality and ethical issues need to be addressed • May only provide information rather than tools needed for behaviour change • May only be effective in the short term • May not be appropriate as a stand-alone method • Difficult to predict engagement accurately

Figure 5.2 The advantages and disadvantages of IT use in health promotion (Koch-Weser, 2010)

Overview of advantages

The previous pages have discussed in some detail Internet application advantages, computer-based applications and mobile phones, including the integration of theory and the interactive nature of IT. In addition to these findings, health interventions that utilise online resources or applications have the potential to teach a number of people who would not usually be targeted or may not usually seek health information through the traditional channels (Buller et al., 2001). Seeking IT-based health information can be empowering; there are opportunities for building social networks, emotional support and sharing experience through the use of the Internet (Korp, 2006). A study by McCoy et al. (2005) proposes that the Internet has potential for self-management education and to promote long-term behavioural change for physical activity and diet, which if true may have potential for the reduction of other lifestyle-related diseases. A study that examined the use of a diabetes risk calculator found that those who had calculated their risk as highest (via entering data on exercise, diet, lifestyle or BMI) were more likely to spend longer looking at the information on a website. Those at increased risk of developing type 2 diabetes mellitus were interested in learning more on the subject both through interactive features and through reading materials suggesting the

 potential to reach *at-risk groups* (Holmberg et al., 2011).

Overview of disadvantages

The digital divide refers to the fact that the 'well educated and well off have access to and use the Internet to a much greater extent than those who are less well educated and who are less well off' (Korp, 2006: 82). Income and education both feature strongly within the notion of the 'digital divide'. The digital divide is not just a country divide, or developed versus developing countries, as this divide can exist within countries. In the UK, for example, around 79% of the highest social classes use the Internet in any location compared to 34% in the lowest social classes (MORI, 2005).

It is possible to hypothesise the problems that some users may face based on the profile of users. For example in the Wyoming Rural AIDS Prevention Project – an Internet programme for MSM – it was observed that completion of the programme was associated with income, accessing the intervention at home, time to load screens and finding navigation easy (Williams et al., 2010). This may suggest that those who did not complete the programme were only able to access the Internet away from home, had lower levels of IT skills and less time to work through the intervention.

Consideration of the reasons why populations access the Internet may also need some attention. For example, Jones and Biddlecom (2011) note that adolescents used the Internet on a daily basis, but few considered it a main source of information about contraception or abstinence. Groups were more likely to rely on and had greater trust in traditional sex education sources such as school, family members and friends. This might suggest that the Internet is not always a solution for achieving a health goal, despite the advantages (e.g. discussion of sensitive issues may be easier and younger age groups are more likely to have competent IT skills).

According to Korp (2006), the Internet may also promote anxiety in some aspects of health, alongside fostering a narrow definition of health. By focusing on individual aspects of a person's health, the Internet is not encouraging inclusion of wider societal influences. The Internet also promotes vested interests (e.g. pharmaceutical companies) of groups who reinforce the medicalisation of health with an emphasis on profits rather than the wellbeing of the individual.

A health practitioner has goals which include education about health issues, enhancing health behaviour or empowering individuals, all of which may be contradictory to commercial websites. Websites can be created for profit or designed for commercial purposes, promote unhealthy behaviours or contain inaccurate information.

Diversity is an important concept for health promotion practice that should not be neglected in the enthusiasm for working with new forms of IT in health. 'Language proficiency, race, culture and other socio-cultural differences may not be acknowledged' (Cashen et al., 2004: 210) and may make health promotion through IT inappropriate or ineffective when working with diverse groups. Cashen et al. (2004), for example, note that patients with low literacy are less likely to use the Internet and other e-health applications, and traditional broadcast media are still an important information source for some groups and especially those with lower education levels. Information should be made more accessible for those who have the greatest need for information, not just the majority. This may mean designing information for low literacy levels, in different languages and in different formats in order to reach diverse groups. (Chapter 3 has more information about working with hard-to-reach groups.)

ACTIVITY 5.4
Designing a website

You are working for an organisation that targets homeless people and you want to design a website that encourages healthy behaviours and practices and facilitates access to services (e.g. social services) among the homeless, who, by the nature of the group, have limited resources.

1   What sort of topics might you want to cover?
2   How would you enable access to the website for this group?
3   What potential problems can you identify using this method with this group (look at Figure 5.2 to help you).

USING INFORMATION TECHNOLOGY IN HEALTH PROMOTION

Kreps and Neuhauser (2010) argue that effectively designed communication should have the reach of mass media and the impact of interpersonal connections. This would suggest a selection of techniques that use sources with wide reach such as the Internet alongside techniques that facilitate access to IT combined with elements that promote interpersonal communication such as social media, feedback mechanisms such as interactive quizzes or other forms of interaction. This sounds potentially difficult for practitioners who may not be familiar with IT. Not all IT applications require the health practitioner to be an experienced IT user. As a health practitioner, designing resources is an essential part of IT use. The next section will cover tailoring health promotion materials through IT and designing resources through a series of design steps. The following section will also consider alternative ways to involve IT in health promotion. The health promotion remit extends wider than developing resources and health practitioners may also have a role in encouraging appropriate use of e-health applications. Internet advocacy (as opposed to media advocacy) may in addition be a way to achieve the wider societal goals of health promotion practice.

TAILORING INFORMATION

One advantage of using IT is the potential to include a 'tailored' element. Tailored information is information that is adapted for individuals and is usually matched to characteristics. This might be social factors such as demographics and/or psychological factors such as beliefs or attitudes (see also Chapter 2). In IT messages can be tailored to individuals rather than a general population more easily than using traditional media (Suggs, 2006). There is room for integration of theoretical constructs into messages, and this can mean that information is more relevant to an individual person or group of people (see Case Study 5.2). The Health Development Agency (HDA, 2004) suggest that targeted and tailored information demonstrates evidence of success in interventions while reinforcing the suggestion in Chapter 2 that information can be matched to a clearly identified target group. Evidence tends to predominately suggest that tailored information does show some benefits over non-tailored information. Stretcher et al. (2005) highlight the strengths of web-based tailored support materials in conjunction with nicotine replacement therapy (NRT) over a non-tailored cessation programme. Other research notes the impact of individually targeted messages in increasing positive attitude changes (Langille et al., 2011).

Case Study 5.2

Tailoring messages to theoretical models

The transtheoretical model (TTM) has been used in tailoring information to a number of health behaviours. The five stages of change that were specified in Chapter 1 are: precontemplation (not interested in change), contemplation (thinking about change), preparation (preparing to change), action (performing the change) and maintenance (maintaining the change).

An example of how the model has been used to tailor messages to those at different phases of change can be illustrated as follows. In smoking prevention the information might be tailored to each stage: those in the contemplation phase might be given a message that says: 'Do you know there is a range of help available to you to help you quit?' Or those in the action stage might be given a message that says 'Well done – you are doing really well at being smoke-free.'

ACTIVITY 5.5
Tailoring messages

You are designing part of a website for encouraging physical activity, based on the TTM. Users answer a series of short questions and once they have submitted these they receive one of five messages aimed at their stages of change based on the TTM. This message is designed to encourage those who are exercising at low levels to increase their exercise or to reinforce motivation in those who are exercising at recommended levels.

1   What messages could you tailor to individuals who are at each of the five phases of the TTM? Use Case Study 5.2 to help you.

DESIGNING RESOURCES IN INFORMATION TECHNOLOGY

If health practitioners want to design IT resources in their health communication strategies, a number of key aspects need to be considered beforehand. These include using the target group in the design and development and integrating theory and evidence into practice. Given that IT (particularly the Internet) is competitive and increasingly commercialised, health promotion needs to make sure the information produced has strong design features to compete in the growing global health marketplace. A search of the evidence is essential in providing background information for what should be included in a resource, for example a website. For persons recently diagnosed with HIV, for example, recommendations include providing HIV-relevant information in a stepwise fashion, demographically targeted HIV information and greater utilisation of mobile technology (Horvath et al., 2010).

USING THE TARGET GROUP

In line with Chapter 2, research indicates that incorporating user beliefs into content delivery together with usability testing is vital (McDaniel et al., 2005). The Internet has traditionally been associated with younger users as the presumption is that they are more IT-literate than older adults. McCoy et al. (2005), however, found that participants in their forties and above thought the online delivery of a diet and physical activity programme was not less attractive to older individuals and did not represent a major barrier to participation, thus contradicting previous assumptions. Some studies have also shown that the Internet is a useful tool for reaching the non-traditional users of IT. These examples serve to illustrate that health promotion cannot operate on assumptions, but must involve the target group in the design, development and testing of the resources.

Integrating theory and the evidence base

As outlined in Chapter 1, campaigns should integrate concepts from theory into IT-based campaigns.

The use of the health belief model (HBM) could include tailoring messages to benefits and barriers identified by the user or activities around perceived susceptibility and perceived severity (see Activity 5.6). The use of the TTM could be employed to target different messages at different stages of change (see Case Study 5.2).

ACTIVITY 5.6
Health belief model barriers on a website

The HBM proposes benefits and barriers that are important to health. You are working on a 'look after your heart' website that aims to remove some of the barriers to eating food groups low in fat.

1 List all the barriers you can think of that stop people eating foods that are low in fat.
2 What kind of messages could you give users to try to remove some of these barriers?

Design steps

Lieberman (2001) makes nine recommendations for designing interactive campaigns with young people and adolescents. These include use of appropriate media, use of appealing characters, incorporating challenges and goals, creating functional learning environments, facilitating social interactions, allowing anonymity and involving the target group in design and testing.

Although Lieberman (2001) applied these stages to young people and adolescents, many of these nine phases could be adapted to suit a more general population for interactive campaigns. Young people and adolescent behaviour may be different than adults' in the emphasis on role models and creating of learning environments when adults may already have these skills. However, learning new skills, influencing attitudes or challenging beliefs are important to adopting new behaviours. *Communicating Health: Strategies for health promotion* proposes a similar seven-step formula for general design of IT-based resources (see Figure 5.3). Using appropriate media, role models or credible sources, incorporating goal settings, creating a suitable environment, facilitating social interaction, protecting anonymity and involving the target group should all be included in a website design. This seven-step framework helps to overcome some of the barriers earlier associated with IT (e.g. confidentiality), and makes use of current research to inform design. Although a specialist IT team will be needed in the set-up and maintenance of the website, health practitioners have a role to play in this team by helping to inform the design and content of the site.

1	Include the use of an appropriate medium for that target group For example, older adults may not want to play game-based activities, but may be more interested in using discussion boards.
2	Use role models or creditable sources This could be someone who has performed the behaviour or someone who the proposed target group can relate to.
3	Incorporate ways of goal setting Allow space for people to set goals or targets for behaviour change, supporting these goals as much as the software will allow.
4	Create an environment which is suitable for the topic both in terms of medium used and the style If you are wanting to influence beliefs, a discussion board or real-life stories might be helpful; if you are looking to influence attitudes, some interactive feedback mechanisms might be helpful.
5	Facilitate social interaction Create areas where there is interaction. This could be discussion boards, user stories or ask-a-question areas. Setting up information or forming support networks may help facilitate and support change.
6	Protect anonymity and confidentiality It is essential that mechanisms are in place to allow users to make up their own pseudonyms or to receive email feedback but retain confidentiality.
7	Involve the target group in the design and testing If the target group is involved in the design and testing of the resources and applications, they are more likely to be user-friendly to that group and be used in their intended way.

Figure 5.3 Seven-step checklist for IT-based resources

ACTIVITY 5.7
The seven-step checklist for a website design

You are setting up a website on the Internet aimed at promoting positive body image and increasing self-esteem in women from 25 upwards that will be run by your local health promotion department.

(Continued)

(Continued)

Following the seven-step formula (Figure 5.3), try to answer the following questions:

1 What media sources would you use?
2 What role models or creditable sources might you use?
3 What sort of goal-setting activities might you include?
4 What sort of style would your website adopt (in terms of content, visually, etc.)?
5 How would you facilitate social interaction?
6 How might you protect anonymity of users?
7 Where might you go to get a small sample of your target group to become involved in the design and testing?

INTERNET ADVOCACY

The Internet contains a wealth of information, and given that freedom is something that embodies the ideology of the Internet, there will be information available that can both promote and damage health. Multinational companies, organisations, groups and individuals can all use the Internet and therefore any topic of their choice can be covered. A proportion of these topics can encourage, promote or facilitate behaviours that could impact on individuals or groups in a negative way. Promotion of cigarettes, pharmaceutical drugs, alcohol use or illegal substance use, for example, are products that can be marketed at the Internet user but may in turn have a negative health impact. Tobacco and alcohol promotion can glamorise smoking or alcohol and target younger age groups, and in some countries provide access to these products. It is also a mistake to assume that promotion of unhealthy products is from the companies and promoters only. There are clubs, chat rooms, web pages and websites dedicated to cigarettes, alcohol and illegal substance use run by (and for) those who participate in these lifestyle choices.

The role of the health practitioner must be to compete alongside these messages to make sure that healthy messages also reach populations. Something that is underused but is seeing more and more media attention in a non-health setting is the use of Internet blogs (diary-style Internet-based information) or the creation of clubs, which currently are used by the online community. Ribisl (2003) draws attention to the use of teenage smoking clubs online. The use of Internet blogs and the creation of clubs in health promotion issues are yet to be explored fully. Given that they exist in health-damaging behaviours, the creation of counter-clubs for young people may be a possibility, and Internet blogs of those who are going through a health behaviour change may be a counter-response. Other means of Internet advocacy may be encouraging the use of filters, blocking or regulating technology (i.e. parental control mechanisms) as well as the more difficult task of monitoring health-damaging behaviours.

CONCLUSION

IT has the potential to become part of the global changes in health but generally is considered more effective when it coexists along with more traditional means of delivery. Despite the potential for IT a sense of realism needs to be maintained in order to include those who are unable to access IT and ensure it does not become an easy but ineffective way to reach target groups.

Research into IT is ongoing, and given the array of contradictory or under-researched areas, it will be several years before research is conclusive. By far the best way for a practitioner to proceed is to investigate target groups' preferences; this way communication is more likely to reach those for whom it is designed. It must be remembered that it is not necessarily suitable for all interventions or for all target groups. IT is by no means a 'panacea' to health promotion practice and campaign design, and its use in changing behaviours remains questionable. Current advice suggests using IT if the target group are likely to make good use of the resources available, but in combination with other media and campaign presence.

Summary

- This chapter has considered the advantages and disadvantages of using IT in health.
- It has considered the role of the Internet and mobile phones in detail.
- This chapter has examined the advantage of tailored information via IT, alongside designing resources for the Internet.
- Additional sections have highlighted the role of the health promoter in Internet advocacy and the move to reduce the digital divide.

ADDITIONAL READING

Practical strategies on information technology in campaigns are in Corcoran N (2011) *Working on Health Communication*. Sage, London.

A US-based comprehensive textbook on health technology for health promotion is Bull S (2011) *Technology-based Health Promotion*. Sage, London.

For practitioners that want up-to-date information, regular reading of health promotion journal articles is recommended.

6

USING SETTINGS

NOVA CORCORAN, ANTHONY BONE AND CLAIRE EVERETT

> **Learning objectives:**
>
> - Explore the features, roles and opportunities for the use of a *settings-based approach* in health promotion.
> - Identify disadvantages and problems associated with a *settings-based approach* and consider ways to overcome these.
> - Examine four non-traditional *settings-based approaches* and their potential to promote health.

The settings approach is an established concept in health promotion. Increasing challenges to the promotion of health and the desire to ensure that health promotion is inclusive make debates around which settings to use and how to use them essential. Healthy settings embody the holistic notion of health promotion, as settings recognise that there are wider determinants that can impact on health. People obtain health information from a variety of sources. These include friends and family and stories in newspapers and television, but this still represents a limited selection of opportunities. Clearly, sources of health information need to increase and people need to access a wider range of sources for their health needs. This chapter will examine the role of a *settings-based approach*, highlighting the different contexts that can be used. Four settings have been chosen in this chapter for this purpose.

DEFINING SETTINGS

Settings have received attention in policy documentation at national and international level. The philosophy of healthy settings stems from the *Ottawa Charter for Health Promotion* (WHO, 1986), which emphasised not only the holistic notion of health – that 'health is created and lived by people within the settings of their everyday life; where they learn, work, play and love' (WHO, 1986) – but also the role of healthy environments. This documentation served to highlight the role of settings as a framework where health can be created, promoted and improved in the context of daily lives and routines. The Charter additionally highlights that the responsibility for health promotion should be shared among the community and those who reside in them: individuals, community groups, health professionals, health service institutions and governments. Essentially a settings approach views physical, organisation and social contexts where people are found (Poland et al., 2009).

One of the criticisms of health promotion campaigns in general is that often the behaviour change in question is targeted in a time or place far removed from where the actual behaviour occurs (Phillips et al., 2011), for example sexual health education in a school classroom setting. One of the distinct advantages of a settings-based approach is that the setting itself may be part of the behaviour change process and be able to influence, support and challenge behaviours in a positive way. There is a wide range of settings that can be used in health promotion. One of the first was the worldwide concept of 'healthy cities' that links global initiatives with local action (WHO, 2003). The city can be an appropriate setting to address factors that contribute to the health of different groups. This includes issues around poverty, pollution, sustainable development and social exclusion as well as the support received for health alliances, for example, between public, private and voluntary services.

The current UK government policy document *Healthy Lives, Healthy People* (DH, 2010a) outlines an intention to shift power away from central government and towards local communities, overseen by the new public health service Public Health England. Settings within our communities will undoubtedly continue to feature highly in the future of public health. The White Paper recognises a number of settings as appropriate for health promotion, from GP surgeries and pharmacies through to workplaces and convenience stores.

The settings approach marks a move away from traditional health education to the promotion of holistic health, and has its roots embedded in new public health (Dooris and Thompson, 2001). The move to integrate health promotion and public health together has led to a 'broader investment in structures that lay outside of traditional health service sectors' (Whitehead, 2004) and marks a move away from individual health education towards holistic health promotion. The World Health Organization indicates that settings themselves represent 'practical networks and projects to create healthy environments such as healthy schools, health-promoting hospitals, healthy workplaces and healthy cities' (WHO, 1998: 1).

ACTIVITY 6.1
Types of settings for different target groups

Think of a target group that might benefit from a health promotion intervention.

1 What sort of setting could be used to pass a health message to them?
2 What sort of restrictions could there be on giving a successful health message to this group?

TYPES OF SETTINGS

It has been postulated that a settings approach includes three aspects: a healthy living and working environment, integration of health promotion into daily activities and links with the local community (Baric, 1993). Dooris (2005) indicates that there is no clear consensus on a settings approach, although does propose that it is clear that settings share a number of important characteristics. First, health is seen as being determined by the wider environment. All settings take a broad definition of health whereby individual health is influenced by wider structures of health, rather than a biomedical, narrow definition of health. Second, the setting itself is a complex system of 'inputs, throughputs, outputs and impacts' (Dooris, 2005: 56). Health therefore is part of the wider 'whole' of what an organisation is trying to achieve, be it education, production of a product or financial gain. It is essential to remember that a setting is not a discrete entity, as there are wider factors that can influence a setting in the broader context of society. Third, organisational change and development is important, as for a true settings approach to be taken the organisation often has to evolve or develop to achieve a healthy setting status.

Green and Tones (2011) distinguish between two different types of settings approaches in health promotion. The first approach is health promotion 'in a setting', for example, delivery of an intervention to increase uptake of screening. The second approach is 'using a setting' as a health promotion approach. This takes more of a comprehensive agenda and the setting is utilised in a wider health promotion sphere where environment, policy, interventions or target groups in that setting become part of the whole approach.

Settings allow health promotion to be practised across a broad spectrum and can address the 'whole' problem rather than isolated parts (Whitelaw et al., 2001). This has the advantage of tackling health issues from a holistic angle. Another key feature of settings is that activities can be mutually supportive and do not exist as isolated health issues but can be considered together to create a more coordinated response. Coordination and interaction are at the forefront of a successful setting.

Current ideas in the field of health promotion indicate that a settings approach is not just a delivery mechanism for health promotion as often utilised in the past. A settings approach takes a more holistic approach, incorporating the wider interactions of social, political and cultural movements and influences. Organisations and those who operate within their frameworks are going to be influenced by these variables. The settings approach can only be truly successful therefore when it moves to modifying contexts (social, political, environmental, structural) rather than modifying individuals to improve health. This approach is sometimes referred to as the 'ecological approach' and allows the wider influences of health to be considered in totality. It has been further suggested that developing health policies and an evidence base should also be part of a settings approach (Naidoo and Wills, 2009).

MAIN FEATURES OF SETTINGS

Whitelaw et al. (2001) propose five broad approaches to settings: the passive model, the active model, the vehicle model, the organic model and the comprehensive model (see Figure 6.1).

Models	Setting approach	Brief description	Example
Passive	Neutral setting	Setting offers access to the population and a situation to conduct individual focused activity	Intervention to raise knowledge of World Aids Day via an information stand
Active	Individual focused	Individual focused interventions but includes recognition of wider organisation	Stop smoking programme in an organisation where nicotine replacement therapy is supplied by the organisation
Vehicle	Individual focused and wider context	Setting is the problem, and individual projects can address these	No-smoking policies in a supermarket
Organic	Wider context	Setting is seen as the problem, but individual change is the solution	Office worker seminars for correct use of VDUs
Comprehensive	Entire context	Changing structures or cultures on a large scale via investment, policy, planning, laws, finance	Healthy schools programmes which include a holistic notion of health via changing structures

Figure 6.1 Settings-based models for health promotion, based on Whitelaw et al.'s (2001) model definitions

These five broad approaches can be adopted by the practitioner depending on what is trying to be achieved. Small-scale interventions that aim to raise awareness of a health issue may be part of the passive model. Groups to encourage stopping smoking in a business that are partly supported by the organisation might be part of the active model. Rewriting policies or plans for organisational changes in a supermarket might be part of the vehicle model. Training all staff in the correct use of a VDU (visual display unit, i.e. a computer monitor) might be part of the organic model. Finally, the comprehensive model includes interventions that incorporate wider aspects of health, with organisational changes in policy or practice alongside possible investment or other features that aim to create a healthy 'whole' school or other 'whole' organisation.

ACTIVITY 6.2
Fitting activities to settings-based models

Use the examples in Figure 6.1 to help you decide which settings-based model best fits these activities:

1 Staff training to increase knowledge of discrimination policies.
2 Anti-bullying strategy in a hospital.
3 Staff training for serving intoxicated customers in a pub with new licensing laws.
4 Healthy cities projects.
5 Cookery classes using low fat foods.

It has been argued that for the potential of a full settings approach to be achieved, only the last model (the comprehensive model) fulfils the full holistic criteria. However, given scarce resources, limited budgets, lack of time, expertise and a limited evidence base, the comprehensive model is often unachievable and unrealistic. Therefore this chapter includes the range of all five models as the other settings approaches continue to be implemented and practised in health promotion work.

LOCATIONS OF SETTINGS

A setting can be formal (such as a school or workplace), geographically linked (such as a city) or informal (such as a pub or virtual community). Given the emphasis on policy and settings, some of the first references to settings were healthy hospitals, schools and workplaces (DH, 1992), thereby much of the literature focuses on these formal settings (see additional reading at the end of this chapter). Formal settings include those settings that are more widely used and can provide access to a sometimes easy-to-reach population. These include education venues such as schools and health care services. Literature still advocates that health service organisations retain potential for health improvement that could be expanded (Whitelaw et al., 2012). A number of new uses of hospital settings include accident and emergency departments being used to deliver *brief interventions* around alcohol, which represents an opportunistic approach to settings. Hospitals could be seen as ideal, effective settings because they share similar goals to health promotion (i.e. improving health), they are credible health information sources, utilise existing infrastructures for health promotion such as alliances, networks or planning, and are a point of entry into the health system. They are in a position to provide patient information, prevention strategies and make use of mass media interventions (especially safety or injury prevention). The hospital is also part of the wider community.

ACTIVITY 6.3
Locations of settings

1 Think of as many settings that can be used for health promotion as you can that are formal, geographically linked or informal.
2 Which setting do you think will be the easiest to use? Which setting could potentially have the biggest benefit?

In the UK, the National Healthy Schools Programme (NHSP) provides a good example of a settings-based approach to health promotion. Launched in 1999 as a joint Department of Health and Department for Children, Schools and Families initiative, schools are encouraged to apply for healthy school status based on national quality standards. The programme has criteria for schools to meet under four themes – personal, social and health education; healthy eating; physical activity; and emotional health and wellbeing. A 'Healthy living blueprint for schools' was produced (DfES, 2004) that *supports children in leading a healthy lifestyle and makes the most of resources that already exist*, encouraging schools to play a more active part in shaping attitudes to health and encouraging informed choice. The programme was transferred to the Department for Education in 2011 by the current government and it is intended that the programme will continue to develop in the future along with Healthy Further Education and Healthy Universities although this is still an area of discussion (see later section on healthy universities).

Green and Tones (2011) argue that if a settings approach is to avoid reaching those who are already in a more privileged position, for example those who are employed or in schools, different settings should be considered in order to avoid increasing the gap between the richest and poorest groups. For example, an intervention aimed at those in schools will not reach those excluded from school, and interventions in workplaces will exclude those who are unemployed. They propose that settings should address needs of a wider range of audiences and may have to use unconventional approaches. This means choosing settings for health promotion that are not traditionally used and may be more informal settings. An informal setting may have hard-to-reach populations, use unusual methods or locations and may be one-off. More unusual settings have been used in health promotion over time, for example 'healthy farms'

(Thurston and Blundell-Gosslin 2005). Other settings are used as an ad hoc location, for example in Australia the National Binge Drinking campaign used a large music festival to reach young people (Van Gemert et al., 2011).

THE ADVANTAGES OF USING SETTINGS

There are a number of advantages to a settings approach in general. Dooris (2005) lists a number of these, which include providing a framework to utilise in practice, allowing ownership of health, enabling relationship exploration, recognition of existing initiatives, joined-up working and an awareness of health at all levels. The very nature of settings encourages multidisciplinary and joint working to achieve objectives. The other advantage of settings is the 'normalisation' of aspects of health. For example, if sexual health information was given to everyone in a workplace and discussed in a more open context, this may encourage a growing dialogue of discussion and encourage more people to access sexual health services when needed. It is possible therefore that a setting can offer a 'scale of intervention that matches how most people view the world' (Poland and Dooris, 2010: 287).

There are a number of aspects of the *settings-based approach* that are common to all settings and foster positive steps in health promotion. Peterson et al. (2002) proposes seven elements found to be beneficial to establishing church-based health promotion programmes (see Figure 6.2). Peterson proposes that a strong church-based programme will contain: 'partnerships, positive health values, availability of services, access to facilities, community-focussed interventions, healthy behaviour change, and supportive relationships' (Peterson et al., 2002: 403). Given the broad nature of these seven elements and the nature of the church as an institution, it is equally likely that these seven elements can be applied to other settings, with emphasis on their importance fluctuating depending upon the nature of the setting.

'Partnerships' include collaboration between organisations or the local community, particularly important for sustainability and involvement of key decision makers. Settings are particularly good for engaging participation with stakeholders and promoting joined up working (Poland and Dooris, 2010). 'Positive health values' include the well-known variables of health promotion practice: advocating, enabling and mediating. These three variables need to be engaged to promote health holistically. 'Availability of services' and 'Access to facilities' are needed to enable access to resources necessary in the promotion of health, for example, money, equipment or other spaces. 'Community focused' refers to the value of the wider community who, when included, will be able to assist in providing access and availability to resources. 'Health behaviour change' should include a focus on theory to support any behaviour changes, and 'Social systems support' should be available via networks or groups for supporting change.

Element	Description
Partnerships	Collective collaboration between organisation and other sectors (e.g. church and health professionals, supermarkets, wider community groups)
Positive health values	Advocate, enable, mediate, service, caring. Promote, prevent, education to obtain positive health. Use of organisation for *peer education* to take an active role in health
Availability of services	Wider access to services or increased access to services, across potentially varied populations
Access to facilities	Resources available in the setting (e.g. meeting places, kitchen, exercise spaces) with the needed volunteers
Community focused	Settings should value and include wider community (e.g. volunteers from community)
Health behaviour change	Theoretical concepts are important; desire to change unhealthy behaviours should be included in the setting and supported (e.g. fruit and vegetables at functions)
Social systems support	Social systems support in the setting and in wider community networks (e.g. the surrounding community, schools, offices); the networks should provide support for change

Figure 6.2 The seven key elements beneficial to establishing programmes, based on Peterson et al.'s (2002) elements for church-based health promotion programs

THE DISADVANTAGES OF USING SETTINGS

Currently the settings approach has a limited evidence base (Dooris, 2005), although some areas are more popular than others, with the use of schools in particular attracting a growing evidence base. What should be of consideration in settings are groups who are excluded from that setting. The editor of *Health Promotion Practice* notes in 2010 that there is a greater need for systematic reviews examining the effectiveness of public health interventions delivered in various settings that aim to address the elimination of health disparities (Jack, 2010) emphasising both a settings approach and the potential to reduce inequalities in health through settings.

Settings can be individualistic, exclusive and have practical limitations (Green and Tones, 2011). Health promotion in a settings context should involve everyone in the wider planning process. A settings approach that is centred on a top-down approach tends to be ineffective (Whitelaw et al., 2001). When one (or a small number) of people dictate what will happen, it will be less effective than involving everyone in that setting. Settings that embody this top-down approach neglect the wider context of the setting and will be more likely to exclude or alienate groups. Limited planning, lack of theoretical foundations and poor evaluation mean that interventions will be unsustainable (Bensberg and Kennedy, 2002) and if left unevaluated or poorly evaluated, positive outcomes that have been achieved will never be recognised. An additional variable might be the topics that are selected for the setting. It may be perceived as a good setting, for instance, using nightclubs as a focus for sexual health or alcohol interventions, but those that use the setting may not see it as appropriate or effective. For example, a review of chlamydia screening services suggests that young adults predominately want services offered in traditional health care settings like general practices (Bruga et al., 2011). In addition if subjects are of a sensitive nature confidentiality and privacy may be problematic.

There are a number of practical limitations to a settings approach. These include finance, resources, time, location, staffing or other aspects that influence settings activities. For example, larger, private organisations may have more financial support than smaller, public ones. There will also be other competing priorities, which mitigate against health priorities. The aim of an organisation is not necessarily in line with the fundamental goals of health promotion. If an organisation is concerned with speeding up the production of a product to make more money and the planned intervention requires finance or proposes changes that slow down the production process, health promotion will have to compete with these priorities. The outcome therefore might be that only part of the proposed changes take place, if any at all. Some settings may be difficult to engage, or reluctant to participate. Philips-Guzman et al. (2011) note the fear of negative customer reactions in profit-making businesses to HIV prevention programmes, despite evidence to suggest customers would be supportive of HIV prevention efforts.

A settings-based approach is not perceived favourably to all concerned, particularly if it requires finances, resources or changes which can be difficult, such as structural changes. The settings that tend to incorporate a health promotion framework are more likely to be those that are better set up to deliver and involve others in health promotion – hence schools are a prime example, as few people can argue about the merit of promoting the health of children, and often strong parental or teacher involvement can facilitate the health promotion process.

Whitelaw et al. (2001) argue that problems in the settings-based approach include practitioners undertaking health promotion work with little focus or understanding of working within an organisation but continue to use the label of a settings-based approach. This often has the effect of continuing a limited individualistic approach, which can lead to victim-blaming, alongside the role of the organisation in health promotion being ignored. The wider environment needs consideration to avoid victim-blaming approaches (Bensberg and Kennedy, 2002).

ACTIVITY 6.4
Overcoming disadvantages of settings

Read through this section on the disadvantages of settings.

1   How do you think you could overcome some of these disadvantages if you were using a workplace setting to promote health?

OVERVIEW OF SETTINGS INTO PRACTICE

The four settings that will be examined are: places of worship, universities, personal care (barbers, hairdressers and beauty salons) and convenience stores. The first two have a reasonably strong evidence base supporting their role as an appropriate setting for health promotion. The second two have an evidence base predominately made up of a mixture of a developing evidence-based and 'grey' literature which makes them potentially more challenging to implement. This is not to say that more challenging settings should be ignored in favour of easier settings; if health promotion is to be truly holistic, then more difficult settings will need to become involved in the settings-based movement.

Poland et al. (2009) formulate a detailed framework to help practitioners understand the culture, history and contexts of the setting. This framework has three parts: understanding the setting, changing settings and knowledge development and translation. A series of questions in each part help to plan and implement a settings-based approach. It is recommended that practitioners who are intending to work in settings locate this article to assist in the detail of putting a settings-based approach into practice.

PLACES OF WORSHIP

Opportunities and advantages

Religious organisations and faith groups have often been able to engage in important roles in health (Duan et al., 2005) and thus have potential as a health promotion setting. They can provide a 'promising opportunity to enhance emotional, physical and spiritual health' (Peterson et al., 2002: 401) and 'faith and spiritual beliefs play a role in maintaining health and wellbeing' (Swinney et al., 2001: 42). The role of religious organisations fits with a holistic definition of health, including physical and emotional aspects of health, alongside spiritual aspects of health and the role of a healthy body, mind, soul and spirit which are integral to religious organisations (Peterson et al., 2002). There are numerous examples of the role of religious organisations in promoting health and in the US faith-based organisations have been promoted as being able to assist the surgeon general in the mission to promote health (see Levin and Hein, 2012).

Most research has focused on Christian churches, and has demonstrated that the church is a potentially effective channel for the delivery of health promotion programmes (Resnicow et al., 2002) as well as conclusions that suggest that church attendance correlates with positive health care practices and preventative behaviours (Ayers et al. 2010; Benjamins and Brown, 2004). Advantages can include a strong social support role (Duan et al., 2005) in addition to a tendency to respond to the needs of its community. Religious organisations can influence the health of its members, for example, Swinney et al. (2001) found that church parishioners believed the church has a role in meeting the health needs of its congregation, suggesting there is some expectation that the church will fulfil this role. Markens et al. (2002), in their interviews with pastors of black churches, suggest that pastors also saw health as something that should be promoted through their work in the church community. Therefore the Christian church may be a place where health promotion could take place, where both religious leaders and the religious community may be willing to attend and participate. See Case Study 6.1.

The advantages of using religious organisations are wide-ranging and may allow access to some populations that traditional health promotion efforts may not reach, including specific ethnic groups and older people who may be traditionally low users of health care services. Religious and faith-based organisations have a tradition as being a strong, caring foundation (Peterson et al., 2002) providing financial, emotional or spiritual support in times of need, and tend to be well respected in the community (Reinert et al., 2008). This also gives them the benefit of being a place where social support networks exist. Campbell et al. (2009) note that historically churches and faith organisations have a role that extends beyond spiritual care and are essential partners in the reduction of health disparities. Alongside social support, religious organisations can provide a social life (Christensen et al., 2005) for parishioners as well as a fairly stable congregation who attend over a long period of time. As an actual setting a religious organisation can provide a safe, supportive environment (Peterson et al., 2002) which can help facilitate behaviour changes, as well as the practical resources that religious organisations may have such as kitchens and meeting rooms which may assist in health campaigns.

Role models and credible sources of information in religious organisations include religious leaders. Leaders of these organisations tend to be demographically similar to members, and embody values similar to their congregations (Reinert et al., 2003); it is also likely that given that membership is voluntary, the leaders chosen are viewed as trustworthy sources of information, making them more likely role models. Some research has highlighted barriers to health promotion in this context, for example high religiosity is a significant factor in perpetuating levels of stigma surrounding HIV/AIDS, associating it with a curse or punishment (Muturi and An, 2010), and in other religious organisations prevention of STIs and HIV through condom use is contentious. It is prudent to be aware of any limitations in the context of the religious organisation as each will be different.

Recently, religious organisations have been used for health promotion and health education interventions in a variety of ways, but most commonly to change individual behaviours in relation to lifestyle-related behaviours. Resnicow et al. (2001) undertook an 'eat for life' project in an African American group, and found an increase in fruit and vegetable consumption. Duan et al. (2005) found an increase in uptake after a project to encourage mammography screening among a group attached to a religious organisation. Campbell et al. (2004) undertook the WATCH intervention to encourage colorectal cancer preventive behaviours, which was met with some success as it improved behaviours (e.g. fruit and vegetable consumption) that lowered colorectal cancer risks. Project DIRECT aimed to decrease the burden of diabetes in relation to self-management of the disease, exercise and diet (Reid et al., 2003). Other projects have utilised health workers in the actual setting.

Implications for practice

Campbell et al. (2009) suggest five principles to consider when working in church-based health promotion which can be applied to any religious organisation. These five principles suggest the development of a mutually beneficial relationship and ensuring sustainability are key to progress in developing a settings-based approach:

1   Careful attention to partnership development and building trust.
2   An everything-on-the-table approach to involving churches in recruitment of participants.
3   Efforts to understand the cultural/social context through extensive formative research and involvement of key informants/advisors.
4   An intervention strategy that incorporates the sociocultural environment and can be delivered at least in part by the community.
5   Develop ongoing plans for ensuring programme sustainability (leaving something behind).

The Peterson et al. (2002) framework described earlier (Figure 6.2), which highlights partnerships, positive health values, availability of services, access to facilities, community-focused interventions, healthy behaviour change and supportive relationships, was originally designed for a church setting. Therefore any intervention that utilises this setting could use this framework as a starting point for a settings-based programme designed to promote effective behaviour change.

Healthy body, healthy spirit

Resnicow et al. (2002), in their study 'Healthy body/healthy spirit', targeted African Americans, and the intervention materials involved the parishioners in their design. They used biblical and spiritual messages to reinforce motivation. The design of an 'eat for life' cookbook included recipes submitted by the church group. Other resources followed a spiritual and religious theme. For example, videos included biblical and spiritual themes to motivate healthy eating and an audio cassette designed for performing exercise to gospel music combined with spiritual messages to match the length of the workout routine.

Case Study 6.1

ACTIVITY 6.5
Designing messages for a religious organisation

1   Choose a religious organisation or faith group.
2   Based on the ideas in Case Study 6.1, what other resources could be designed to promote health using a spiritual message in a religious group?

Religious organisations with strong leadership roles are more likely to sustain projects in the long term. Research suggests longevity of the church indicates sustainability of projects, as does the active membership size (Duan et al., 2005). Christensen et al. (2005) found that religious organisations with stable, consistent leadership are the most likely to express interest in a health-related programme for cancer prevention, and competing priorities were the most likely reasons for refusal. They also found that smaller organisations were the most interested in a cancer prevention programme, suggesting perhaps fewer competing priorities.

Points to consider

There are gaps in the literature on religious organisations and their role in public health (Christensen et al., 2005). There is a distinct African American US focus in many studies, leaving other groups missing from the research (Christensen et al., 2005; Peterson et al., 2002). Bopp and Webb (2012) highlight the potential role of mega churches (congregations with 2000+ members), although their research indicated that ministers' roles in health-related activities had to compete with other church activities. This is a possible avenue for future research. A limited evidence base for health promotion and health education work utilising other faith groups means that other religious groups, such as Muslim or Sheik groups, are not evident in the literature. This has some implications for research, given that it is unclear whether different places of worship – mosques or temples, for example – are appropriate settings to promote health. Poor dissemination of results and few controlled designs also mean that the evidence base remains patchy (Peterson et al., 2002).

Despite barriers, religious and faith-based organisations still hold great potential for reducing health disparities and promoting health in their members and are an underutilised setting for the promotion of health on a small and large scale. If health promotion is truly to achieve health for all, and access some of the harder-to-reach groups, particularly older age groups and some ethnic minority groups, a variety of religious organisations will need to be included within health promotion frameworks.

UNIVERSITIES

Opportunities and advantages

Universities have a key role to play in the promotion of health of those working and studying within their walls and for the wider community. Changes to fee structures and current demands on university spending mean that universities strive to meet higher delivery expectations, quality, demographic changes in those attending universities and higher costs. The increased student tuition fees that have followed the Browne Report (Browne, 2010) will impact further upon these challenges and institutions will need to become better, more competitive and more efficient than ever before.

Universities were not originally included in the first concepts of the 'settings' approach to health (Dooris, 2001; Whitehead, 2004) and there has been a lack of international or national standards around health-promoting universities. However, the Health Promoting University initiative was launched in 1995 by the University of Central Lancashire and in 1998 the WHO published a working document, highlighting that 'the settings-based approach to health promotion can potentially enhance the contribution of universities to improving the health of populations' (Tsouros et al., 1998: 3).

The UK government document *Choosing Health: Making healthy choices easier* (DH, 2004) highlighted the importance of integrating health into the organisational structures of universities and colleges. The DH and Higher Education Academy then funded the National Research and Development Project on Healthy Universities (Dooris and Doherty, 2009). Recommendations for the development of a National Healthy Universities Framework were submitted to the DH in March 2010 and a decision is currently awaited. Health-promoting universities that do exist have often adopted a student-centred approach, most commonly running campaigns involving students via the student union (Dunne and Somerset, 2004). The Healthy Universities approach places emphasis on whole system involvement and interaction, and targets improvements for students and staff alike. Within this whole university approach, the student union remains an obvious choice for health promotion work. It is in close contact with the health needs of its members because its officers are elected and are drawn from the client population so the needs are known at first hand. The health agenda is also appropriate to settings; for example, advice about the stresses of student life including financial, welfare, sexual health and other health-related topics.

Although whole university approaches have been slow in coming, there are few reasons why universities should not be key health promotion settings. They share similar characteristics with other educational facilities, for example schools and workplaces, both of which are highlighted as appropriate health promotion settings (DH, 2004). Universities tend to be large organisations employing a variety of staff (academic and non-academic, technical, research and others) and are in a good position to promote the health of students (Dunne and Somerset, 2004) and staff. Dooris and Thompson (2001) consider that universities are well placed for a settings-based approach to health promotion for a number of reasons, including: their focus on education, training and research, a role in developing and creating innovation, and the fact that universities are a community resource.

University of Central Lancashire

The University of Central Lancashire is one of the first UK-based universities to embody the health promotion settings approach. It is now part of the healthy universities network (www.healthyuniversities.ac.uk) with a number of other institutions. The healthy university initiative aims 'to integrate within the university's culture, processes and structures a commitment to health and to developing its health-promoting potential and to promote the health

Case Study 6.2

(Continued)

(Continued)

and well-being of staff, students and the wider community' (UCLAN, 2006). To achieve this, a variety of initiatives have been put into place in the university setting. These include new policies (corporate health policy and transport policies), student and staff health-related information (health handbooks, sexual health projects) and changes in the curriculum and research to encourage health in other non-health disciplines. (UCLAN, 2006)

Implications for practice

In order for universities to become healthy settings the drivers behind the university relating to the environment of the setting, the core business of the setting and connections to the wider community need to be understood (Healthy Universities, 2011). Ultimately a university is a business and understanding the structures can help to aid healthy settings approaches. The healthy university toolkit provides a range of case studies and ideas for practice and suggests that implementing the healthy university approach includes designing campaigns and integrating health promotion methods alongside maintaining 'three balancing acts'. These three balancing acts are:

- Combining high visibility innovative action with a commitment to leading long-term organisational and cultural change.
- Enabling wide-ranging stakeholder involvement while securing senior-level commitment and corporate responsibility.
- Anticipating and responding to public health challenges while explicitly helping to deliver the core institutional agenda.

These 'balancing acts' mean that university settings approaches should be developed to recognise that health could be part of a wider taught curriculum, e.g. climate change campaigns across a range of subjects (geography, media studies, etc.) alongside the university priorities of teaching, learning and increasingly profit making and business organisation (see also Case Study 6.2).

ACTIVITY 6.6
Designing a healthy university campaign

The Healthy Universities website suggests the following ideas for health campaigns. Within a university context, health promotion campaigns can take a variety of forms, including:

- One-off half day or full day events on a particular subject, such as healthy eating, alcohol or mental health – including food taster sessions, information stalls and interactive activities.

- Sustained campaigns focusing on a particular subject or an array of different subjects over a longer time frame.
- These campaign ideas can be supported by a wide-ranging communication programme or strategy utilising different types of media appropriate to the setting.

1 Using the toolkit for guidance, how would you go about designing and implementing a project that aims to reduce STIs. Think about the whole context of the university. The toolkit is available at www.healthyuniversities.ac.uk/toolkit/uploads/files/communicating_health_messages_guidance_package.pdf

Points to consider

Dooris and Thompson (2001) highlight a number of challenges to a health-promoting university. These include organisation, ownership and different setting perspectives. Organisation can be difficult, for example, where to locate the project(s). If it is to include the whole university a student/staff split should not be evident, which makes it more difficult to choose the location. Implementation depends on cooperation, both internal and external (Xiangyang et al., 2003). Project ownership is another challenge; for example, the whole university should be involved in managing and working towards sustainability, although this may be difficult to achieve without initial leadership. A different settings perspective may be shared by different staff and students. Potentially controversial topics such as workloads or working conditions may be considered inappropriate, yet if the university is to take a wide settings approach these topics will need to be included in an initial address. Evaluation also needs to be added to the planning process. Long-term measurement can be difficult, especially if different cohorts of students are being measured. Full-time students traditionally take three or four years to complete their programmes, and measurement may involve another cohort, making generalisations difficult.

Universities have the capacity to change and a 'responsibility to educate and influence the next generation of decision makers and managers' (Dooris and Thompson, 2001: 156). Healthy universities need to evolve in their creation of national and international standards to enable all the good work achieved by 'healthy schools' to continue into adulthood education.

PERSONAL CARE SETTINGS

Opportunities and advantages

The evidence base is not widely available on the use of beauty salons, barbers and hairdressers as a setting for health promotion but it is growing. This is not due to lack of projects in these areas, rather that there are a number of small-scale projects ongoing that are not incorporated into the evidence base, and the available evidence can mostly be found in research that makes up the body of grey literature. There is some support for these settings; the Department of Health's Sex Worth Talking About campaign (DH, 2009b) recognised that beauty salons and barbers can play a role in STI prevention, designing a contraceptive advice leaflet tailored to those attending   hair and beauty salons titled 'Your style, your contraception; You've got more options than you think'. Health promotion worldwide has been using salons, barber shops and hairdressers to promote health in a variety of other ways. For example, Lewis et al. (2002) report on the Barber and Beautician STD/HIV Peer Educator Programme, where local barbers and beauticians educated clients about STIs and HIV and distributed condoms and educational materials.

ACTIVITY 6.7
Using barbers or beauty salons

Choose either barbers or beauty salons as a setting.

1   What sort of health promotion topics could be covered in this setting?
2   What are the disadvantages of using this setting? How might you overcome these?

Given the nature of other personal care settings, they could have the potential to deliver interventions at a wider level. Linnan et al. (2001) propose four levels – intrapersonal, interpersonal, organisational and community – which could be delivered via the beauty salon (and similar) settings (see Figure 6.3). Interventions on an interpersonal level could include publicity material available at the reception desk or waiting areas. Organisational interventions include using wider aspects of the settings, for example, introducing policies designed to promote health to the whole salon or studio environment. Community-based interventions include those which involve the wider community, for example, the setting becoming an educational resource for the whole community.

The North Carolina 'BEAUTY and Health' pilot study (Linnan et al., 2005) indicated that cosmetologists delivered cancer prevention messages around a number of cancer-related key topics (designed in conjunction with the stakeholders in the programme). The cosmetologists continued to deliver these messages up to 12 months after the pilot intervention, with more than half of the customers reported to have visited their health care providers since the study, indicating the feasibility of cosmetologists and beauty salon owners in health promotion delivery interventions.

Interpersonal	Publicity material with health messages including leaflets, posters, flyers, videos or information booklets. Interaction between more than one person (e.g. client and care provider) including discussion, one-to-one or question/answer.
Organisational	Policies or interventions on a wider scale in the salon setting (e.g. healthy food or drinks for clients or no-smoking policies).
Community	Involving community in design or implementation of an intervention (e.g. becoming an education resource for the whole community, being involved in whole community activities). See BBHOP case study.

Figure 6.3 The multi-level interventions in a personal care setting

Beauty salons have the advantage of being women focused, with frequent attendees. A reasonable time period is spent there (30 minutes upwards), where a wide range of topics are discussed between client and cosmetologist (Linnan et al., 2001). One important topic to focus on is the link between beauty and health (Linnan et al., 2001), and the salon environment is already set to discuss these issues (Linnan et al., 2005). This represents a promising setting for maximising reach, reinforcement and the impact of public health interventions aimed at addressing health disparities, as a study among African American women has shown (Linnan and Ferguson, 2007).

Women attend beauty salons with a motivation to look attractive or beautiful, therefore health promotion plays an important role in achieving this goal. Solomon et al. (2004) also propose that the social environment in a beauty salon encourages conversation, information giving and advice, with several conversations leading to health topics, and often there are displays in salons that promote healthy messages, for example healthy eating. The salon is a feasible and desirable setting to introduce health promotion messages, given the health topics that cosmetologists say they discuss with their clients (Linnan et al., 2005). For example, eating fresh fruit and vegetables with their vitamin and mineral properties are linked to strong nails and good hair quality.

Barber shops have always been traditionally male-dominated environments. Barbers are a location where men gather to enjoy each other's company and can be sources of entertainment or conversation, including facilities such as television, games or videos (Lewis et al., 2002). This indicates that time may be divided between self-care and leisure. There is evidence to suggest that there are successful small-scale initiatives which use barber shops. Linnan et al. (2011) highlight the potential of barber shops for increasing physical activity, and work by Releford et al. (2010a, 2010b) focuses on CHD. For example the Black Barbershop Health Outreach Program (BBHOP, 2012). BBHOP is aimed at African American men, and volunteers in barber shops screen for diabetes and hypertension and promote lifestyle-related changes and recommendations to prevent cardiovascular disease (Releford, 2010a, 2010b) (see Case Study 6.3). Other examples use a more informal approach; *Barbershop* is a magazine written by the Central Lancashire Primary Care Trust's (PCT) mental health race equality team, which focuses on mental health issues in a magazine style format (Improvement and Development Agency, 2011).

Barber shops

The Black Barbershop Health Outreach Program (BBHOP) focuses on diabetes, high blood pressure and prostate cancer. This campaign works in partnership with community, state and private organisations in barber shops across the US. For example in May 2012 the focus was in California and they offered free diabetes and blood pressure screening in approximately 100 black owned barber shops. This setting is also used for 'P.E.P. Talks' (prostate education project) which men at risk can access. More information is available at http://blackbarbershop.org/.

Points to consider

There are a number of creative programmes utilising beauty salons and barbers, but few are evaluated effectively for their impact. The evidence base for using personal care settings is limited, despite the potential role of these locations to promote health. The grey literature has projects that run worldwide, and there is growing focus on. Making these projects available using the Internet as a dissemination tool. Future practice should aim to undertake well-planned campaigns in these settings, with clear evaluation frameworks to encourage best practice.

Not all topics are suitable for these 'open' and sociable environments, and some clients may not consider it appropriate to discuss some health topics, especially more sensitive subjects. However, it is clear that some topics, such as healthy eating, sensible drinking or stopping smoking, have a role to play in appearance and could be good topics for this setting. The salon or studio environment is accessed by a range of clients and customers who should be included in the design of projects to enable their future success.

CONVENIENCE STORES

Opportunities and advantages

There is growing interest in food retailers for promoting health especially in the area of diet and nutrition. McCormack et al. (2010) note the potential of farmers' markets and community gardens to increase fruit and vegetable consumption and availability as well as the potential for revitalising neighbourhoods. Glanz and Yaroch (2004) examined grocery store initiatives for environmental policy and pricing initiatives to increase fruit and vegetable intake and note the potential of these for improving health. In 2008 the English government launched the Change4Life scheme, with the aim of encouraging families to improve their diets and activity levels. One area identified in the scheme, of particular relevance to the settings approach, is access to healthy food and snacks in deprived areas. It is recognised that access to fresh fruit and vegetables can be limited in low income areas where convenience stores are the main setting for food purchasing (DH, 2010b). Following the Healthy Living Neighbourhood Shops project in Scotland, which successfully increased sales of fresh fruit and vegetables by 30% during its pilot (NHS Health Scotland, 2007), the English Convenience Store Programme worked with shops to position fruit and vegetable displays and chilled cabinets in prominent positions, and to use the Change4Life branding to promote these foods (DH, 2010b).

The Buywell Retail Project

The Buywell Retail Project ran from March 2009 until March 2010 as a pilot project in 15 convenience stores in deprived areas of London. The scheme aimed to improve access to fresh, affordable and sustainable fruit and vegetables. It did this by providing each store with an individual store development plan, business support, fresh produce training, Change4Life marketing materials and a launch event. Evaluation showed an average 60% increase in fruit and vegetable sales across the stores. See www.sustainweb.org/ buywell/ for more information.

Case Study 6.4

The initial phase of the Change4Life Convenience Stores Programme involving 17 stores provided extensive intervention, including provision of a chilled cabinet part-funded by the scheme and considerable support from a project co-ordinator. The cost to the Department of Health of this high intervention was approximately £5100 per store. In the next phase of the project, during which the scheme was rolled out across 74 further stores, intervention costs were decreased to an average of £300 per store. It is also noted that although the increases in fruit and vegetable sales indicate the scheme has been successful, the value of fruit and vegetable sales as a proportion of total sales remains very small. Future evaluations may be advised to consider the intention of shoppers when purchasing fruit and vegetables from convenience stores, for example, whether items were bought in place of confectionery as a healthier snack, or bought to use in main meals at home. This may assist with future development of similar schemes. See Case Study 6.4 for an example scheme.

ACTIVITY 6.8
Settings and convenience stores

The Change4Life Convenience Store Programme has also developed links between shops and local schools and cooking clubs to further promote healthy eating and cooking skills.

(Continued)

(Continued)

If you were working with stores in the scheme:

1   What other interventions could you use to promote sales of fruit and vegetables in
    the stores?
2   What methods could you use to ensure that the fruit and vegetables are eaten after
    purchase, so that people are encouraged to continue buying them?

Points to consider

There is no correct way to undertake opportunistic health promotion, apart from
the fact that it should reach those targeted through an opportunity to make healthy
choices easier when shopping for food. Materials are less likely to have the potential
to be tailored, but should still follow designs suggested in previous chapters. In
convenience stores, the production of recipe cards to be given away free to shoppers
can be placed near the fruit and vegetable sections, but could additionally be placed
by the ready meals to attract the attention of shoppers who would perhaps not
usually visit the fresh produce section.

The additional promotion of existing public health resources and networks, such
as Change4Life, in these store locations or on the recipe cards is likely to further
enhance the impact of the scheme. By providing this health information in a practical,
relevant but opportunistic setting a wider target audience will be both reached and
influenced.

CONCLUSION

Dooris (2005) argues that there is still a lack of evidence base for a settings
approach. This is partly due to the focus on single factors, for example one disease
or risk, in the settings approach. He argues that the application of theoretical-based
evidence to a settings approach is needed alongside decision makers who are
engaged in the planning and evaluation levels (Chapter 7 considers *evidence-based
practice* in more detail). When undertaking settings-based activities, the evidence
base should be examined as thoroughly as possible, including the grey literature (see
Chapter 7). One common principle shared by the research in settings is the
partnership approach to development, which suggests clear involvement and
engagement of target groups in the design and delivery of programmes. Settings
encourage a bottom-up approach that needs to be maintained throughout campaign
development. Using a setting may provide access to an entire community, but this is
not to say that everyone in that community will want to be involved; finance, time,
resources, disinterest are all obstacles which will need to be overcome or worked
with. 'It is becoming increasingly clear that twenty-first century problems can only

be meaningfully tackled through adopting holistic and comprehensive approaches within the places that people live their lives' (Dooris, 2005: 63). Health promoters of today should be constantly seeking to adopt comprehensive approaches in tune with wider population needs.

Summary

- This chapter has highlighted the role of the settings-based approach in health promotion and has defined settings and their characteristics.
- This chapter has considered their advantages and disadvantages.
- This chapter has explored four settings in health promotion. These include two large settings, religious organisations and universities, alongside two smaller settings, personal care and convenience stores.
- The merits of these settings to promote health were highlighted together with their challenges to the promotion of health.

ADDITIONAL READING

An interesting chapter on the settings-based approach can also be found in Green J and Tones K (2011) *Health Promotion: Planning and strategies*, 2nd edition. Sage, London.

A framework for implementing a settings-based approach: Poland B, Krupa G and McCall D (2009) Settings for health promotion: An analytic framework to guide intervention design and implementation. *Health Promotion Practice* 10 (4): 505–516.

See also the Healthy Universities toolkit and website at www.healthyuniversities.ac.uk.

7

EVIDENCE-BASED PRACTICE

NOVA CORCORAN AND JOHN GARLICK

Learning objectives:

- Explore the role of evidence-based practice in health communication.
- Examine the application of evidence to health promotion interventions via a number of mechanisms.
- Identify problematic areas of evidence-based practice and consider ways to overcome these.

Health communication interventions now frequently use evidence-based practice to enhance the likelihood of successful outcomes, although this has not curbed the lively debate around evidence-based practice. The appropriateness of using evidence in health promotion, the types of evidence to use alongside the applicability and transferability of this evidence to practice are all sources of ongoing discussion. On the one hand, health practitioners are being continually reminded that evidence-based practice is important to health promotion and health education work, and there is a growing evidence base accordingly. On the other hand, they are being urged to exercise caution when applying the available evidence to their work. This chapter will examine what evidence can be used in health campaigns, and the potential problems that can arise from utilising the evidence base. Acceptability and transferability of evidence will be explored, alongside how to establish and use the evidence available in practical work.

DEFINITIONS OF EVIDENCE-BASED PRACTICE

Evidence in health promotion campaigns and its use in practice has received a mixed reception, with arguments ranging from health promotion success being wholly reliant on demonstration of a strong evidence base, to arguments that suggest health promotion and evidence are incompatible (McQueen, 2000). The 51st World Health Assembly urged all member states to 'adopt an evidence-based approach to health promotion policy and practice, using the full range of quantitative and qualitative methodologies' (WHA, 1998). Recent authors postulate that evidence is imperative to health promotion practice, and de Leeuw (2011: 1) notes that evidence is the 'Swiss army knife of empirical understanding'. Evidence is evident in nearly all decisions about health and healthy lifestyles even if it is not explicitly recognisable. For example the decision to restrict sun-bed use to over 18s only and the additional law that states all tanning salons have to be staffed from April 2011 was predominately made a legal requirement based on evidence. This evidence came from research highlighting the dangers of sun-bed use, i.e. a report commissioned by Cancer Research UK, and subsequent data from the *British Medical Journal* among other sources (Cancer Research UK, 2009).

Speller et al. (2005) propose that in evidence-based health promotion practice attention needs to be paid to four activity areas. These are: systematic review of research and collation of evidence; developing and disseminating evidence-based guidance; developing the capacity to deliver evidence-based practice; and learning from effective practice. This suggests there remains a gap in health promotion as to what works best in relation to incorporating evidence into practice.

The premise of *Communicating Health: Strategies for health promotion* is that for health communication to be successful there is a need to look at evidence critically and apply what works in order to demonstrate effectiveness. Given that health communication has a variety of aims, this includes to justify decisions that have been made, to evaluate effectiveness or efficiency of an intervention, or to justify resources, time or funding.

An evidence-based approach is one that 'incorporates into policy and practice decision processes and the findings from a critical examination of demonstrated intervention effects' (Rychetnik and Wise, 2004: 248), or as proposed by Wiggers and Sanson-Fisher (2001), the systematic integration of evidence into the planning process of health promotion activities. Evidence-based practice is about making sure that an intervention is supported by evidence, enabling the design of a successful intervention (Harrison, 2003). There are a number of different ways that the words 'evidence-based practice' have been used. In the area of public health, Harrison (2003) divides these into three categories, which can be adapted to health promotion practice (see Figure 7.1).

In health communication, the practitioner will usually make use of 'the evidence base for public health' (or health promotion), to either make evidence-based policy and practice decisions or utilise the evidence to inform their own policy and practice.

1	**Evidence-based policy and practice** Practice that attempts to use current evidence to make a judgement or decision on the most appropriate intervention(s).
2	**Evidence-informed policy and practice** A situation where evidence (usually a wide range of evidence) has been used to inform an intervention.
3	**The evidence base for public health** This includes the whole catalogue of evidence available for public health interventions, policies or practice and can be used by practitioners to inform their practice.

Figure 7.1   Three categories of evidence-based practice

RATIONALE FOR EVIDENCE-BASED PRACTICE

All practitioners working in health communication should be aware of the current evidence base that informs best practice. There is increasing recognition of the importance of evidence-based practice that can be used to justify health promotion activity (Green and Tones, 2011) and an agreement that health promotion programmes 'should be based on clear and rigorous evidence about their efficacy' (Harrison, 2003: 229).

The rationale for using the evidence base is strong. It has been argued that there is an ethical imperative to employ evidence so that health promotion does no harm (Green and Tones, 2011). This theme is also taken up by Raphael, who argues that ethical health promotion practice requires clear recognition of the 'ideologies, values, principles and rules of evidence' (2000: 355). Another important reason is the move to close the gap between theory and practice, alongside increased confidence of practitioners that the decisions they have made are the correct ones. Green and Tones (2011) suggest a triangulation approach to evaluation and suggest decisions should be based on the best available evidence at that time. Wang et al. (2005) also agree that evidence-based practice in public health should mean that health care decisions are based on the best evidence available.

Current ideas would suggest that unless multidisciplinary areas such as health promotion and public health utilise the evidence base, practitioners will continually have to defend decisions that have been made without evidence. While other disciplines around health promotion are using evidence, for example medicine and physiotherapy, health promotion is in danger of becoming a discipline that cannot prove that interventions are cost effective, reliable, valid or acceptable unless it starts and continues to incorporate elements of evidence-based practice into all areas of its discipline. Kreps (2012) argues that if practitioners are slow to use evidence to accomplish health promotion goals, and due to the complexities of health communication, strategic guidance from evidence is essential to ensure success.

ACTIVITY 7.1
Evidence-based practice rationale

1 Can you think of any other reasons why evidence-based practice might be important to health promotion practice?

Rychetnik and Wise (2004) propose two questions to consider when using an evidence
base in health promotion. First, is the evidence relevant and useful to current policy
and practice contexts, and second, what is the reviewer's role in (a) interpretation and
(b) advocating action based on that interpretation? Green and Tones (2011) suggest
that with evidence the question should go beyond the fundamental 'does it work'?
Other components should be examined including: how it works, the outcomes,
context, replication, appropriateness and acceptability. In addition practitioners need
to consider a 'systematic and reproducible approach' (Brice et al., 2011) to data
collection to avoid timewasting and missing key research.

Advantages of using the evidence base in practice can ensure that time, money,
people and resources are directed effectively. Tang et al. (2003) propose that
interventions often will find it difficult to obtain policy support if they do not have
evidence of effectiveness. Green and Tones (2011) also argue that evidence can
provide some back-up resistance and support for proposed policies or programmes
that practitioners may not agree with.

WHAT EVIDENCE CAN BE USED?

The concept of evidence-based practice implies a rational, logical or sequential
concept, starting with problem identification, moving to selection of intervention,
then implementation (Harrison, 2003). Rarely are the processes so simple. One of the
difficulties is extracting the relevant research to solve the problem to assist in the
formulation of programme design. Hill et al. (2010) notes difficulties in defining
problems, locating information to solve these and conducting relevant literature
searches as tasks a health practitioner needs to demonstrate competence in.

It has been argued that only randomised control trials (RCTs) or systematic reviews
should be used to inform the evidence base in health promotion, alongside the use of
observational studies (Wang et al., 2005). Speller et al. (2005) argue that this focus
on RCTs has weakened health promotion's position in policy and has a tendency to
equate wrongly lack of evidence with lack of effect. There are a number of reasons
why health promotion does not always lend itself to an RCT. For example lack of
resources mean that not all aspects of health can be tested in this way and it only gives
a partial overview of the problem being identified, particularly when an intervention
includes social or economic conditions. Literacy, acceptability, appropriateness, lack

of resources, time and funding in addition to lack of trained staff can all impact on an intervention that attempts to be replicated in another area. Fortunately, more recently it has been recognised in public health practice that evidence is generally a result of the more complex interaction between evidence from research (such as systematic reviews) alongside other sources and includes judgements that are centred around local area resources, circumstances and ethical implications (ECDC, 2011).

It is a challenge to health communication campaigns to find evidence that is relevant to the topic area and avoids the reductionism notions that pervade the evidence base. The move to develop an evidence base through clinical practice has been heavily supported through government and medical organisations. Unfortunately this enthusiasm has not been replicated in health promotion. However, growing practical experience is increasing the notion of 'best practice' in health promotion and leading to more success (Nutbeam, 1999).

The more traditional uses of evidence through clinical trials are not the only source that health practitioners can use. Tang et al. (2003) propose four classifications of evidence that could be used in health promotion (Figure 7.2).

1	**Evidence that meets scientific fact criteria**, i.e. replicable, proven or repeatable over time
2	**Evidence that has success and can be predicted**, but can only be replicated at local level in a certain time frame and only then if resources or certain settings are available
3	**Evidence that has success but does not meet causality criteria**, but can be repeatable
4	**Evidence that has success and can be predicted**, but does not meet causality criteria and can only be replicated at local level in a certain time frame and only then if resources or certain settings are available, and thus universal application is not achievable

Figure 7.2 Four classifications of evidence used in health promotion, based on Tang et al. (2003)

Tang et al.'s (2003) classifications in Figure 7.2 illustrate four main classifications of evidence. This ranges from evidence that meets 'scientific' facts, to that which can be replicated under certain conditions, to evidence that is repeatable, but not controlled. Finally, there is evidence that is successful and can be predicted, providing it is applied to local levels if it meets certain criteria and conditions.

ACTIVITY 7.2
What evidence do you use?

1 Using Figure 7.2 to help you in your health promotion work, which category of evidence do you use the most? Alternatively, if you are a student in a health-related programme, which evidence have you used the most for your assessments?

The NHS Centre for Reviews and Dissemination (2001) provides a similar hierarchy of research evidence that can also be used in health care practice. Wiggers and Sanson-Fisher (2001) place this into a number of levels.

Figure 7.3 illustrates the levels of evidence that could be included in health campaigns. Clinical decision-making tends to be based on level 1; at least one appropriately designed RCT. However, health promotion will frequently find itself using levels 3 and 4; large comparable differences within time or location, and opinions of authority groups, descriptive studies or reports. This is often because the evidence simply does not exist at the higher levels (1 and 2), but also because health promotion fundamentally takes a holistic view of health and some health topics do not fit comfortably under the heading of a randomised control trial. Whatever figure we choose to favour, Figures 7.2 and 7.3 serve to illustrate that health promotion interprets a wider picture of health (not just the clinical trial-related one) and therefore most practitioners will use a combination of evidence from a number of levels.

Level 1: At least one appropriately designed randomised control trial
Level 2a: Well-designed controlled trial without randomisation
Level 2b: Well-designed cohort study
Level 2c: Well-designed case control study
Level 3: Large comparable differences in time/location with/without the interventions
Level 4: Opinions of authority groups with clinical experience, descriptive studies and reports

Figure 7.3   Levels of research evidence, based on Wiggers and Sanson-Fisher (2001)

ACTIVITY 7.3
Planning with evidence

You are planning a community-based project in a small local neighbourhood to try to reduce theft and mugging in the area, which is unusually high. The residents identify poor street-lighting and nothing for 'youths' to do as the problem. The local council proposes community police officers as the solution. There are no RCTs or systematic reviews demonstrating the link between any of these solutions (street lights, 'bored' youths or community police officers) to the problem.

1   What do you think you would do to address the issue?
2   What evidence do you base this on?

Like other health interventions (e.g. clinical practice), health promotion is made up of a linked ladder of activities, with national policies at the top, down to individual health promotion programmes at local level. The basic question of evidence-based practice – 'Does it work?' – may be posed at these different levels. Collecting evidence 'is the end result of processes for filtering, reviewing and synthesising research studies' (Marks, 2003: 6), something that requires skill and practice. There are a number of sources available to the health practitioner to enable access in evidence-based practice.

WHERE TO FIND EVIDENCE

Electronic bibliographic databases

Electronic bibliographic database use is on the increase among health practitioners via access to the Internet. Practitioners can make use of databases that have a focus on clinical, public health and health promotion issues such as the Cochrane Library, which publishes systematic reviews of information, and the Campbell Collaboration, which contains evidence on randomised trials, interventions and evaluations.

Electronic or paper journals

Electronic or paper journals are another way of finding information for evidence-based practice. The *British Medical Journal* (*BMJ*) was one of the first databases to appear online with free access. There are a large number of national and international journals available in the areas of health promotion, health education and public health. For example, Oxford journals publish journals online including *Health Education Research*, *Health Policy and Planning* and *Health Promotion International*. Other journals include those that are designed to be accessed online. Biomed central (www.biomedcentral.com) is also a good source for open access journals especially for global issues. The US-based PubMed website is an excellent source of journal abstracts and some free text articles (ww.ncbi.nlm.nih.gov/pubmed).

Government and other organisation documentation

Governments in the developed world are usually well resourced to be able to access, collect and codify evidence in health and health care areas of activity. In the UK the National Institute for Health and Clinical Excellence (*NICE*) produces evidence briefings as well as providing new reviews and the development of guidelines, interventions and technology appraisals of further health-related topics. In early 2012 there were 36 dedicated public health evidence-based briefings, along with a range of other evidence briefings relevant to different areas of health-related practice. Topics include physical activity, unintentional injury, prevention of cardiovascular disease, maternal and child nutrition, smoking cessation, school-based interventions, tuberculosis, STI prevention and harmful drinking. Those in development include oral health, hepatitis B and C, workplace health and domestic violence. Case Study 7.1 has an example of diabetes guidance.

Preventing type 2 diabetes NICE example guidance

Preventing type 2 diabetes: population and community-level interventions in high-risk groups and the general population. Public Health Guidance PH35 (NICE, 2011).

- Ensure healthier lifestyle messages to prevent non-communicable diseases (including type 2 diabetes, cardiovascular disease and some cancers) are consistent, clear and culturally appropriate.
- Address any misconceptions about the risk of diabetes and other non-communicable diseases that can act as barriers to change. This includes the belief that illness is inevitable (fatalism) and misconceptions about what constitutes a healthy weight. Also address any stigma surrounding the conditions.
- Ensure any national media (for example, television and online social media) used to convey messages or information is culturally appropriate for the target audience.
- Messages and materials should: – highlight the need to reduce the amount of time spent being sedentary – highlight the importance of being physically active, adopting a healthy diet and being a healthy weight – increase awareness of healthier food choices, and the calorie content and nutritional value of standard-portion size meals and drinks.

ACTIVITY 7.4
NICE evidence base

Visit www.guidance.nice.org.uk/PHG/Published. What documentation is available in this section that could be used to help you design small- or large-scale health promotion campaigns in your area of interest?

Despite the emphasis on, and effort directed to, the collection of the best available evidence, there is also recognition within government that the best may be the enemy of the good. In an internal paper, NICE (2005) questioned the rigid application of hierarchies of evidence. It focused on the question of whether it was more important to implement a recommendation based on high-quality evidence rather than one supported by a lower level of evidence, regardless of the effect, size or other factors that may determine its impact on health. As a result it was decided that NICE would no longer publish the classification grade of the evidence which supported its guidelines and recommendations. In effect, NICE would be able to decouple its assessment of the quality of its evidence from the importance of its recommendations.

UK government publications also recognise that in some specific areas there may simply be no 'good' evidence to work with. In the NICE evidence into practice briefing on promotion of physical activity (Cavill et al., 2006), it is suggested that there are areas where it is not possible to suggest review level evidence-based actions or interventions, such as: physical activity intervention studies with people from black and ethnic minorities and physical activity intervention reviews among people with physical limitations. However, in both cases experienced practitioners in the respective fields were able to identify a number of themes of enquiry.

Grey literature

Grey literature refers to informal published material, which by its nature does not fit into a clearly identifiable group. This can include local reports such as those produced by NHS groups or Primary Care Trusts (PCTs) and conference proceedings. The use of local needs assessments, health impact assessments (HIAs) or community profiles may help in identifying problems from a qualitative prospective. Networks may also be available where practitioners can share ideas.

Grey literature can be difficult to find and has been described as the proverbial needle in a haystack (Matthews, 2004). However, useful material can often be found on the websites of relevant organisations and, increasingly, databases of grey literature are being established. An example of such a database is the Library of Grey Literature maintained by the West Midlands Public Health Observatory, some of which is publicly available. Users of grey literature will need to satisfy themselves of the quality of documents accessed unless specific information is available on quality criteria checking.

ACTIVITY 7.5
Grey literature

1 What grey literature could you use in your work?
2 Have you compiled any materials that could be counted under the 'grey literature' heading?

PROBLEMS WITH USING THE EVIDENCE BASE

Although there are many positive uses and justifications for evidence-based practice, there are also a number of problematic areas with the application of evidence, in particular in the discipline of health promotion. First, evidence alone cannot constitute good practice. Tang et al. (2003) argue that evidence can inform practice, but not produce practice. Without skilled practitioners who are able to find, locate and apply the evidence, interventions will be unable to fully utilise the evidence base.

Another issue is that the relevance of evidence for a practitioner depends on the quality of the evidence and how it can be implemented (Green and Tones, 2011). Not all evidence is applicable to practice, in particular the use of some of the more traditionally proposed evidence bases (for example, RCTs). Traditional evidence and the theories or models of health that it is based on (in particular the biomedical model) may not be appropriate in the application to health promotion (Raphael, 2000). Health promotion supposes a holistic definition of health and operates in a context of social, political and environmental influences, which much traditional evidence may have ignored. Evidence also is inclined to include a distinct Western bias and material from a non-Western perspective is sparse (McQueen, 2000, 2002). Application to groups who are non-Western therefore may be difficult or inappropriate.

Developing countries can be particularly problematic; some countries have less well-established evidence bases and may rely on other countries for evidence. Economic, social or political environments may be more complex in these areas, with less funding or resources available (Overseas Development Institute, 2006). But does this imply that evidence-based health promotion is simply a creation of the West, which has nothing to learn from the experiences of developing countries? McQueen (2000) reports the proceedings of an ad hoc group of attendees at the Fifth Conference on Global Health Promotion in Mexico City in 2000. He proposes that in the context of prolific debate on health promotion evidence in the Western world, there was a clear lack of participation from those representing the experience of the developing world. Underlying reasons for this exclusion were:

- The conduct of the debate in the English language by Europeans and Americans, or others educated there; and
- A restriction on participation in the debate largely to the academic elite or those privileged to hold the type of government office that allows involvement.

The ad hoc group thought that the 'missing voices' should be uncovered and the evidence from developing nations brought into full play. To support this aim a set of recommendations was made. These include establishing a working group, incorporating unpublished materials, consideration of alternative evaluation methods, alongside representation of a multicultural working group.

ACTIVITY 7.6
Including developing countries

Read the recommendations for including developing nations in research again.

1   What problems can you foresee in following these recommendations?
2   How could these problems be overcome to include developing nations into evidence-based practice?

There have been some examples of the inaccurate use or misreporting of evidence. Cummins and Macintyre (2002) cite the example of 'food deserts' where some ideas have been replicated as fact, even though they might not be true. They refer to these facts as 'factoids'; imagined or speculated facts that become true. Health practitioners are encouraged not just to assume evidence is true, but to question facts.

Some evidence can be very difficult to translate into practice, and McQueen (2002) suggests that lack of detail in relation to transferability can hinder the application of evidence-based practice to health promotion. It has also been argued that it may be unethical to wait for evidence from actual local settings. If there is a major public health issue (e.g. infectious disease such as H1N1) that needs to be addressed quickly, the wait for evidence can be lengthy and it may be necessary to act without a fully developed evidence base (ECDC, 2011).

It is possible that the term 'effectiveness' may need some thought. For example when indicators are developed for campaigns they may not always demonstrate appropriate outcomes. Macdonald and Davies (2007) argue that effectiveness may need to be considered in a different way for health promotion. For example, they consider measurement in complex programmes such as school-based interventions and propose conventional indicators or behavioural outcomes (i.e. mortality rates) may not be the most appropriate way to measure interventions, instead suggesting input proxy measures (such as teaching sessions) and intermediate proxy indicators (such as attitude change), This may help to develop a broader picture of outcomes in the short term.

ADAPTATION AND TRANSFERABILITY

Implementation is an important part of using evidence-based practice (Newman and Harrier, 2006). Health promotion practice sometimes has difficulty translating the evidence base into a practical programme, so even if the evidence exists replication may be unclear. There is little point of a study advocating good practice if a practitioner cannot then replicate this. Evidence-based practice should be able to be replicated in a different place and a different time (Harrison, 2003). One of the problems with this is that interventions are often population- or location-specific and are difficult to replicate in a different context. Transferring evidence to 'local circumstance, local capacity, local ownership and local obstacles to implementation' (Marks, 2003: 23) is a challenge for health practitioners.

There has been some interest in the problems associated with applicability of evidence in evidence-based practice, alongside some of the factors associated at local levels that impact on transferability (Sharp, 2005). Card et al. (2011) suggest that in order to select suitable evidence a variety of questions could be asked of the evidence. They suggest a seven-step framework for adaptation. This includes:

- Does the intervention have behaviour/health status goals that are relevant for the new target group (e.g. increasing condom use may not be appropriate in all target groups)?
- Does the intervention show strong evidence of having achieved its goal?
- Does it address determinants of behaviour (e.g. attitudes, intentions) that are relevant and acceptable to the new target group?
- Does the intervention use methods that are appropriate for the new target group?
- Does the implementing agency have access to the resources needed for adaptation to the new target group?

An alternative series of criteria is applied by Wang et al. (2005) to see if the intervention is acceptable and transferable to current practice. They propose a practical approach to getting evidence-based findings into practice in different contexts via a series of acceptability and transferability questions.

Each question covers key areas that may make the difference between success and failure in health promotion practice. Figure 7.4 allows the selection of a study, where the practitioner can then ask a series of questions to see if that study can be successfully replicated in practice. This does not guarantee instant success as wider variables may mitigate circumstances, but it does go some way to covering the pitfalls associated with the replication of others' work. Wang et al. (2005) propose that after the questions in Figure 7.4 have been applied, there are likely to be four outcomes. First, that the intervention finds little difference between the study setting and the target setting and the intervention will demonstrate health outcomes should it be implemented. Second, the intervention could meet the requirements with additional work, for example, some minor adjustments to the original study. Third, there may not be enough evidence to apply transferability or applicability information, and more research is required. Last, there may be a considerable difference between the study group and the target group, and the application of the study is inappropriate. Another approach should be adopted in this instance, either by working towards implementation of the study at a later date or by choosing another approach to the problem. See Case Study 7.2 for an example.

Applicability	
1	Does the political environment allow this intervention? Are there any political barriers to implementation?
2	Would the population accept this intervention? Does the intervention go against any social norms or ethical principles?
3	Can the contents be tailored for the intervention group?
4	Are there resources to implement this intervention?
5	Does the target group have sufficient educational levels to understand the intervention?
6	Which organisation will provide this intervention? Are there barriers in this organisation to implementing this intervention?
7	Do the providers have the skills to deliver the intervention?
Transferability	
8	What is the baseline prevalence of the health problem? What is the difference between the study setting and the target setting?
9	Are the characteristics similar between the study and the target population? Will demographics such as age, socioeconomic status, etc. impact on the effectiveness of the intervention?
10	Is the capacity to implement the intervention comparable between the study and the target area in political environment, acceptability, resources, delivery structure and skills of providers?

Figure 7.4   Questions to ask in determining applicability and transferability, based on Wang et al. (2005)

Case Study 7.2

Applicability and transferability design

Bones in Mind was an osteoporosis programme run by the Woman's Institute (WI) with Cornwall and the Isles of Scilly Health Promotion Department in a predominately white, rural area. This programme trained a number of older women from the WI to deliver a 10-week programme. The 10-week programme was attended by members of the local WI in the local area. The women in the groups ranged between 40 and 70 years. The WI provided the local halls and refreshments for the sessions. Training, publicity materials and other costs were paid for by the local health promotion department. The sessions ran once a week for two hours and included weight-bearing physical activity regimens, nutritional activities and advice. Informal evaluation indicated that women were more likely to eat calcium-rich foods and partake in physical activity at follow-up, compared to when they first joined the programme. (Cornwall and the Isles of Scilly Health Authority, 1999)

ACTIVITY 7.7
Applicability and transferability

You are working for a local health promotion organisation. Your target group is: women 30–50, in an inner city area, predominately Asian and white, some of whom are non-English speaking. There are some local women's groups who have expressed an interest in an osteoporosis programme, but your health promotion department has no additional funding to help you. You do have access to a physical activity coordinator who usually works with children and who is willing to help you.

Look again at the 'Applicability and transferability questions' in Figure 7.4.

1 Can you apply the Cornwall and Isles of Scilly Bones in Mind (Case Study 7.2) osteoporosis programme to the new target group?
2 Is there anything you might need to do to make sure the programme is successful?

HOW TO ESTABLISH AN EVIDENCE BASE

One of the problems with application of an evidence-based approach is the lack of evidence available. Harrison (2003) argues that this difficultly arises because different disciplines and practices contribute different approaches, analysis or collection to the evidence base. One of the main problems for health communication is that findings from intervention studies seldom report in depth the processes of intervention development. Barretto et al. (2010) highlight three reasons why this information would be useful for practitioners:

- It would help guide the development of new interventions and refinement or revision of existing ones.
- It would provide a framework and methodology on which other health practitioners and researchers could build.
- It would increase transparency of the development process and enhance the interpretation of the intervention's effects.

One of the roles of a health practitioner is therefore not just to utilise the existing evidence base, but to apply consistent methods to practice, and to add other evidence through practice to inform future health promotion work. Harris et al. (2012) highlight a range of ways that practitioners and researchers should be involved in the dissemination of evidence-based practice, including encouraging practitioners to be involved in collecting and discussing evidence.

Nutbeam (1999) highlights four ways that best practice can be achieved (see Figure 7.5) and thus lead to providing evidence of effectiveness. He suggests that if these processes are in place, there will be greater success of objectives and thus the intervention. Alongside this there will be a greater likelihood that the intervention will be able to be added to the existing evidence base, and thus inform future practice.

1	**Analyse** epidemiological, behavioural and social research in planning the intervention
2	**Use established theories** that are appropriate to the intervention planned to develop the programme
3	**Ensure that conditions are favourable** for the intervention, including resources, training, services, capacity, etc.
4	**Implement the intervention in a sample** of suitable size and sufficient duration to enable results to be identified over other variables

Figure 7.5 Four ways that best practice can be achieved, adapted from Nutbeam (1999)

According to Figure 7.5, the first way best practice can be achieved is through the analysis of epidemiological, social or other research to assist in the planning of the intervention. This means using evidence-based policy and practice – as Harrison (2003) suggested – to make a judgement or decision on the most appropriate intervention(s). The second way of ensuring best practice is to use established theories (Chapter 1 provides a detailed account of ways to use these theories). The third way is to ensure favourable conditions. Supportive environments and conducive conditions, together with well-stocked resources, are more likely to herald success. Last, the intervention should be implemented over a large enough sample and for long enough duration to enable results to be demonstrated that can be attributed to the project and not to other variables, for example, another project. By following designs for best practice, the likelihood of a successful intervention that can be replicated by others is higher.

USING AN EVIDENCE BASE TO IDENTIFY METHODS AND STRATEGIES

'Turning evidence into practice depends on the quality of evidence, its accessibility, effective methods for dissemination, and a context which favours implementation of effective interventions' (Marks, 2003: 4). Evidence that is available for health practitioners covers a wide range of areas, and a health practitioner working in the areas covered should be aware of the evidence base for their particular line of work. The reviews themselves can cover good practice, methods that work best in target groups, strategies to reduce certain aspects of health-related problems and other key evidence for successful health promotion work.

Newman and Harrier (2006) propose that one of the most important things a practitioner must do in using the evidence is to ask questions. They provide a list of ways evidence could be used, based on research by Sackett et al. (1996). Some of these questions are applicable to health promotion practice. These include using evidence to identify:

- Causes of problems;
- Goals or aims of interventions;
- Ways to reduce occurrences of ill health;
- Ways to improve health; and
- Perceptions of others (e.g. the target group).

Sometimes causes of problems need to be identified to be able to highlight issues to focus on. For example, perhaps young people smoke because they want to impress their peers, or think it makes them look 'cool'. If this, or other reasons for smoking, can be identified, interventions can focus on the 'causes'.

Evidence for message design

A study by Longfield et al. (2011) suggests that future messages about safer sexual behaviour should do the following: emphasise consistent condom use with all types of partners, improve knowledge and correct misconceptions about HIV/AIDS, STIs and condom use.

1   If you had to choose one area to focus on for a campaign, which one would you pick and why? Think about what you have learnt throughout this chapter to help you support your answer.

Case Study 7.3

Formulation of goals, aims or objectives can be taken from evidence-based research. Evidence-based practice should be able to provide some suggestions of ways to overcome ill health or improve health which can be adapted for practice. And finally, evidence can give practitioners perceptions and ideas about the proposed target group that can support their own work with the target group.

One of the most straightforward ways to identify appropriate interventions or target groups from evidence is to utilise recommendations from national organisations. The NICE Internet database contains a large number of recommendations and guidance, as highlighted earlier. In the area of maternal and child health, NICE has made a number of recommendations for practice. These include the recommendations listed in Figure 7.6 (NICE, 2008). Health practitioners, policy-makers and other health professionals are encouraged to put into action these recommendations. As a health promoter, this may mean selecting one or a combination of these recommendations for practice and tailoring guidance accordingly.

Maternal and child nutrition evidence
Provide information on the benefits of a healthy diet and give practical, tailored advice on how to eat healthily throughout pregnancy.
Inform women with a body mass index (BMI) over 30 about the increased risks to themselves and their babies. Encourage them to lose weight before becoming pregnant or after pregnancy.
Provide a structured, tailored programme of ongoing support that combines advice on healthy eating and physical exercise and addresses individual barriers to change. Do not recommend weight-loss during pregnancy.
During the booking appointment, offer information and advice on the benefits of taking a vitamin D supplement during pregnancy and while breastfeeding.
Provide breastfeeding information, education and support in a setting and style that best meets the woman's needs. In the last trimester of pregnancy, run an informal group session focused on how to breastfeed effectively.

Figure 7.6   A selection of edited evidence from NICE (2008) maternal and child nutrition

ACTIVITY 7.8
Evidence and maternal and child health

Read the edited recommendations from the NICE (2008) maternal and child nutrition in Figure 7.6.
   You are a health promoter working in the area of maternal and child health and have a small amount of money to spend on a nutrition-based project.

1   Based on the evidence, identify a target group and setting and outline campaign ideas that you could undertake which would cover some of these recommendations.

Practitioners should critically appraise health promotion literature to enable interventions to be informed by the evidence base. Wiggers and Sanson-Fisher (2001) propose that practitioners should examine literature critically to determine four things: reliability, validity, acceptability and sensitivity. Thus practitioners can ask questions of the research under these four headings.

   Rada et al. (1999) propose that intervention information in health promotion comes from two main sources: the target population and research based on other populations. To ensure that health promotion interventions are successful, the information required should come from both sources. To gain information about the target population it is probable that sources may include: local morbidity or mortality statistics, community profiles, needs assessments, interviews/focus groups or other forms of local information. Undertaking these processes can be represented as a circular model that a practitioner can move through before achieving the final result (see Figure 7.7).

The basic steps in Figure 7.7 demonstrate the stages a practitioner could move through to incorporate evidence-based practice into health promotion work. These are simplistic steps, but they give an idea of at what stage evidence is used in the planning and evaluation processes. This model illustrates the fact that evidence is reviewed and analysed throughout the intervention process. When the intervention is complete it is evaluated, and these findings (either successful or unsuccessful) are then fed back into the evidence base for the next health promotion project.

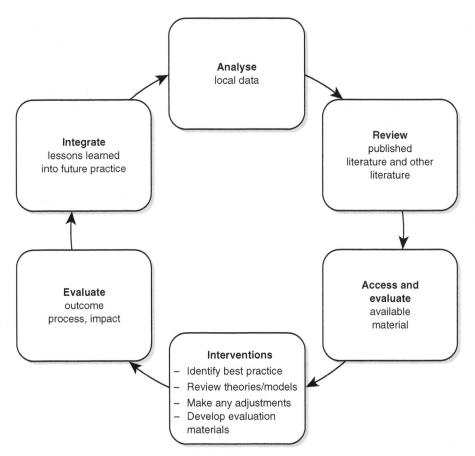

Figure 7.7 The steps for inclusion of evidence-based practice, based on Levandowski et al. (2006)

CONCLUSION

Health promotion should be in a position to promote and enable access to the evidence base, particularly when IT allows wider access to materials. Marks (2003: 28) argues that 'the key to evidence-based practice . . . is that the evidence base and review of effectiveness of interventions should be accessible and useful to decision makers'. This includes practitioners in non-Western countries who have been excluded or overlooked previously. Those who need evidence should be able to access what they need to make informed choices and decisions., Evidence should be accessible to those who need it and the evidence itself needs to have characteristics which allow practitioners to adopt evidence for practice such as guidance on ways to implement evidence in practice (Sharp, 2005).

The debate about the use (or non-use) of evidence-based practice should be taking a back seat to more productive discussions around the well-trodden grounds of the problems of using evidence. If practitioners want skills to implement and access evidence, why can they not be gained? (After all, the job of most health promoters is, to some extent, to give skills and knowledge to others.) If evidence is not readily available – why is it not available? How can it be made more easily available? Other essential topics should include ways to move forward strategies to compile, use, apply, transfer and implement evidence-based practice into health promotion planning and programmes. Only when we see action will we start to see change.

Summary

- This chapter has highlighted the role of evidence-based practice in health promotion practice.
- The debates and issues surrounding the use of evidence and the current debates on evidence-based practice have been highlighted.
- An applicability and transferability framework has been explored and applied to practice.
- Ways to establish and utilise evidence-based practice, including accessing evidence for practice and building up the evidence base in health promotion, have been examined.

ADDITIONAL READING

Fink AG (2012) *Evidence-Based Public Health Practice*. Sage, London.
A text that covers a range of issues.
Earle S, Lloyd CE, Sidell M and Spurr S (2007) *Theory and Research in Promoting Public Health*. Open University/Sage, London.
A book that considers the relationship between theory and practice.
The National Institute for Health and Clinical Excellence (NICE) provides guidelines for practitioners including evidenced-based briefings and public health guidance in the UK. This is available at www.nice.org.uk.

8

USING EVALUATION

SUE CORCORAN

Learning objectives:

- Explore models of evaluation theory in relation to communication processes in health promotion programmes.
- Apply theoretical models of evaluation to the practice setting.
- Identify strategies that would be required to plan an effective evaluation of a health promotion communication programme or campaign.

Evaluation can be defined simply as determining the value or assessing the worth of something. It has an important role in health promotion and is central to the development of a robust evidence base. Evaluating communication in health promotion can be challenging and it requires the practitioner to have an awareness of the range of evaluation methods available and to apply these to the chosen project with appropriate rigour. Communication in health promotion by its nature is not rigid and sometimes cannot be measured by traditional scientific methods. This requires the practitioner to be flexible when considering the evaluation tools and methods. The bedrock of health promotion evaluation is a four-stage model of formative, process, impact and outcome evaluation. This chapter explores evaluation in relation to communication processes within health promotion programmes and campaigns with an emphasis on the need for a multidimensional approach. It also considers methods to employ when evaluating outcomes to stakeholders. Examples of good practice are included as well as opportunities to test out the theoretical knowledge base.

DEFINING EVALUATION

Evaluation can be described as: 'A systematic, rigorous and meticulous application of scientific methods to assess the design, implementation, improvement or outcomes of a programme' (Rossi et al., 2004). In health communication evaluation the methods used can be quantitative and qualitative, formal and informal. In general all these methods will be used as the nature of health promotion is by definition an art and a science which enables people and communities to discover the synergies between motivation and optimal health (O'Donnell, 2009). At one level it will be incorporated into a practitioner's day-to-day activity and on another level it will be systematic, rigorous and may be undertaken by outside researchers.

Health promotion as a discipline is concerned with empowering individuals to take control and influence their own health. Providing evidence through evaluation requires the use of methods that reflect health promotion goals. Health is not just a physical entity but a resource for everyday life. Evaluation is a complex process and cannot answer every question it poses. It is therefore important that the planning is clear from the outset so that when unpredictable outcomes are identified there is a mechanism to explore them. An evaluation to ascertain whether nurse telephone triage only reduces emergency ambulance use may demonstrate that it does not. This would be seen as a service failure. If however the service was evaluated in terms of whether it reduced walk-in hospital emergency department attendances it might be deemed a success (Brophy et al., 2008).

There are numerous reasons why health promotion programmes and activities should be evaluated. Figure 8.1 illustrates the reasons for evaluating using four main headings, namely, fiscal, quality, evidence and policy. All these areas will need to be considered when undertaking evaluation and will influence the understanding of the potential and limiting factors for success to enable improvement in future health promotion practice.

ACTIVITY 8.1
Who is interested in evaluation and why?

You want to evaluate a campaign 'Dancing for Health', a twice-weekly dancing programme for adults. Its aim is to improve the physical and mental health of people who live on a large social housing estate in a city.

1 Make a list of the people and organisations who would be interested in the outcomes of the campaign.
2 Using Figure 8.1, which headings might be appropriate to an evaluation of the campaign?

Reasons for evaluation	Examples of evaluation
Fiscal	Ensuring cost-effectiveness Influencing allocation of resources Securing funding for current and future projects Legitimising budget reduction Enabling economic analysis
Quality	Assessment of need Assessing effectiveness against existing standards Using performance indicators Recognising ethical dimensions to research and campaigns Ensuring accountability Using clinical governance to inform practice
Evidence	Increasing the evidence base Developing theoretical concepts Improving methodologies Sharing experiences Understanding limitations
Policy	Informing future planning Influencing and legitimising policy Gaining political capital Assisting in the development of long-term strategies

Figure 8.1   Twenty reasons for evaluating health promotion programmes, adapted from Katz et al. (2000) after Downie et al. (1992)

WHY EVALUATE COMMUNICATION IN HEALTH PROMOTION?

All health promotion occurs within the context of communication. The nature of communication has changed and there is more emphasis on people actively seeking and exchanging health information using available technologies such as social media, websites and mobile devices. Abroms and Lefebvre (2009) describe the success of Barak Obama's presidential campaign where new technologies were used extensively and their relevance to public health campaigns. Communication is seen as dynamic where information sources and those receiving them interchange roles. It is therefore important that extensive evaluation is conducted into finding out what the audience's needs are and how they respond to and process the messages (Rimal and Lapinski, 2009).

Opportunities for using different approaches for the dissemination of health promotion activity make it increasingly important to develop a reliable evidence base across all health disciplines. Hills and McQueen (2007) note in a critique

>> of the Ottawa Charter (WHO, 1986) that it scarcely mentions the importance of measuring the effectiveness and impact of health promotion programmes. The acknowledgement that health *inequalities* exist in all societies has been well documented. What is less known is how to improve the health and wellbeing of all people regardless of their life chances. In identifying the nature of health inequalities and its effect on health communication it is important that those working in the field of health promotion and public health acknowledge this important tenet when using evaluation tools. The House of Commons Health Committee report (2009) emphasised that the current lack of evidence and evaluation of large public health programmes was unacceptable. It stressed that without the appropriate information the tackling of major health inequalities will remain complex and challenging.

OVERVIEW OF MODELS AND THEORIES OF EVALUATION IN HEALTH PROMOTION

The following sections will consider a selection of theoretical models and theories for evaluation in health promotion that are most commonly used for campaigns and programme evaluation. These include the four-stage formative, process, impact and outcome models and including a fifth dimension of dissemination and feedback. Other models that are useful to the practitioner when undertaking evaluation include: economic, pluralistic, participatory, experimental evaluation and social marketing.

Evaluation in health normally involves the bringing together of a variety of assessments which help to define whether an activity has achieved its aims in the short and longer term and describes how the aims were achieved. Evaluation must be integral to the health campaign and not added on later. The evaluation should also continue throughout the life of the activity and beyond, which may constitute months or years in order to ensure that all of the components of the activity are appropriately tested. Sridharan and Nakaima (2011) propose a 10-step approach to evaluation and argue that evaluation should not be formulaic in its design as it will not address the complexity of programmes and that better collaboration between planners and evaluators will be of benefit.

Formative, process, impact and outcome evaluation

The four-stage model of evaluation is widely used in health promotion. As dissemination and feedback are also important to health communication these elements are incorporated to become a five-stage model to make it more appropriate to health communication (see Figure 8.2).

Design phase	Type of evaluation
Pre-testing Needs assessment	**Formative**
Planning, design, implementation and maintenance	**Process**
Immediate effects	**Impact**
Long-term effects	**Outcome**
How successful	**Dissemination**

Figure 8.2   Five-stage model of evaluation

FORMATIVE EVALUATION

Formative evaluation should be undertaken during the planning stage and before the implementation of a programme or campaign. It is also used as an ongoing tool. Some authors will use the term in the same context as process evaluation and this underlines the fact that although models are helpful they need to be seen in the context of everyday activities and that each step in evaluation will diffuse into the other. Formative evaluation involves pre-testing materials and strategies in order to ensure that assumptions made in the planning are examined and addressed. It also helps to prevent valuable resources being wasted. The steps to successful formative evaluation include recognising the scope of the programme and the context in which it takes place. Gaining information from key stakeholders will assist in clarifying the main issues. It is not always easy to ensure objectivity in evaluation if the stakeholder's interests conflict with the aims of the programme. It is helpful to build in an assessment of how different stakeholders respond to different methods, measurements and design (Bryson et al., 2011). See Case Study 8.1 for an example.

Furness Families Walk4Life

Milton et al. (2011) undertook a formative evaluation of a 12-week intervention to encourage walking as a family-based activity. The family unit has been identified as an important mechanism for increasing physical activity. The intervention was undertaken in collaboration with the Ramblers Association. The key evaluation questions were:

- To explore the barriers to walking in families with young children.
- To determine whether partnership working provides an effective approach to walking.
- To determine the appropriateness of the intervention.
- To identify improvements for future implementation.

(Continued)

Case Study 8.1

(Continued)

The campaign offered led walks, telephone support and other tailored resources. Interviews were held with staff who were involved in setting up or delivering the intervention and focus groups were undertaken with participants. The adults reported barriers to success such as the concern about their children's behaviour. It was reported that if families undertook the activities in a group with other families they were more confident and this provided opportunities for social interaction for adults, teenagers and children. The most successful walks were those with a specific destination with an activity at the end as well as things for the children to undertake en route. The outcome of the formative evaluation was that it highlighted the key characteristics associated with delivering a family-based walking programme.

ACTIVITY 8.2
Formative evaluation

You are undertaking a formative evaluation looking at children (aged 10–11) and their attitudes, beliefs, values and barriers to eating fruit and vegetables.

1   What methods could you use to explore these behavioural determinants?
2   How will you extract themes that will help you plan your intervention?

NEEDS ASSESSMENT

Needs assessment determines what the problem is to be addressed in the intervention, how great is the problem and what can be done to meet the need. It is used at the outset of programme planning and is integral with formative evaluation. It has two distinct phases. The first involves consultation with the target group to explore the problem. The second scopes the scale and extent of the issues. Interviews, focus groups and online questionnaires are some of the methods that can be used to explore the problem. The evaluator is looking for behavioural factors such as attitude, values, barriers and benefits which may be used in conjunction with the existing evidence base (Corcoran, 2011).

Consulting communities is a key part of needs assessment and it serves to understand factors that affect health and quality of life. It recognises that health is shaped by individual, social, economic and political frameworks and can engage people and communities in information appraisal, priority setting and the building of future capacity (Smith et al., 2006). Figure 8.3 shows an example of a needs assessment strategy as recommended by NICE (2010).

> **Preventing unintentional road injuries among children and young people aged under 15: Road design and modification.**
>
> **Aim:** To support coordinated working between health professionals and local highways authorities to promote changes to the road environment.
>
> **Action:** provide engineering strategies to prevent injury and to reduce the risk.
>
> **Needs assessment:**
>
> 1 Collect data on injury risk, (traffic speed and volume, etc.). Injuries (level of injury, location of accident, etc.).
> 2 Design measures within local and geographical contexts.
> 3 Take into account all users, e.g. pedestrians, cyclists, car and lorry users, those with impaired mobility.
> 4 Develop an effective process for community engagement.
> 5 Seek the views of children, young people, their parents and carers.
> 6 Seek the views of all interested parties such as emergency services, local businesses.
> 7 Consider changes in the light of overall transport infrastructure.

Figure 8.3 Example needs assessment, from NICE (2010)

PROCESS EVALUATION

Process evaluation concerns the journey taken by the programme. It focuses on all aspects of the intervention. It helps to describe and understand the implementation and contributes to the development of further learning and improved performance. It utilises a wealth of methods that are both qualitative and quantitative and often requires direct contact with individuals or communities. Process evaluation is concerned with whether programme activities were accomplished. See Case Study 8.1 for an example. The Centre for Chronic Disease Prevention and Health Promotion (2009) recommends questions including: How were the messages generated? Was the quality of the intervention maintained? Was the target audience reached? How well were the programme activities implemented? How did external factors influence the programme?

Process evaluation

Reininger et al. (2010) undertook a process evaluation of an obesity prevention media campaign. It aimed to promote physical activity and healthy food choices in Mexican Americans living on the Texas Mexico border. The target population was adult males and females aged between 20 and 64 and their families. The media campaign featured Hispanic role models (i.e. those who had undergone behavioural change) and experts in diet and nutrition who appeared in mass media outlets (morning television and news items) and monthly newsletters. Lay community outreach workers were also recruited.

(Continued)

Case Study 8.2

(Continued)

The process evaluation included:

- Content analysis of media messages and newsletters.
- Monitoring amounts of and locations for newsletter distribution.
- Focus groups with the target population.
- Ensuring that the role models were included and supported in the media campaign.
- Assessing whether the campaign materials were culturally and linguistically appropriate.

IMPACT EVALUATION

Impact evaluation has to answer the question, 'Did it work?' It seeks to track an actual change of status usually within a predetermined time frame. It generally gives stakeholders an indication that the programme is having an impact in the short term. It can be significant when determining issues such as whether knowledge and skills have been achieved or professional practice has changed as a result of the intervention. It may also support evidence for continuation or cessation of an intervention. This is of particular interest for project funders and some stakeholders.

The types of impacts that can be measured in a health promotion programme are shown in Figure 8.4. These include health literacy, social action and influence and healthy public/organisational policies.

Types of impacts that can be evaluated	Descriptors of impacts
Health literacy	Improved health-related knowledge, attitudes, motivation and confidence. Behavioural intentions and personal skills concerning health lifestyle. Knowledge of how to access health services.
Social action and influence	Community participation and empowerment. Social norms and public opinion.
Healthy public policies and organisational practices	Implementation of policy statements, legislation or regulation, resource allocation, supportive organisational practices, enhanced engagement with health communication programmes.

Figure 8.4 Types and descriptors of impact, adapted from the Australian Institute of Primary Care (2008)

ACTIVITY 8.3
Impact evaluation

A needle exchange programme for drug users has been deemed effective after undertaking an impact evaluation.

1   What do you think might constitute an effective programme when measuring the impact of a programme of this nature?
2   What would the impact evaluation not tell you?

OUTCOME EVALUATION

Outcome evaluation describes the effects of a programme over a longer period of time. Knowledge and skills of individuals can be measured, but in outcome evaluation the application of these follows a continuum influenced by changes in health behaviours, expectations of health and socioeconomic factors. The effects are often measured by indicators such as quality of life, *equity* of access to services, disability, morbidity or mortality Thesenvitz et al. (2011) suggest that there are four levels of audience for longer term outcomes.

- *Individual*: To initiate or maintain personal behaviour change.
- *Networks* (e.g. family and friends): The social environment that impacts on behaviour.
- *Organisations*: The development of policies and procedures.
- *Society*: The making of laws.

ACTIVITY 8.4
Well Man clinics

Well Man clinics have been set up in 10 GP surgeries in a low socioeconomic area in Scotland. The target population is men between the ages of 40 and 65 years. The clinic offers monitoring of blood pressure and weight and cholesterol levels. It records smoking, alcohol and drug use and discusses lifestyle issues such as diet, sexual health and exercise.

1   What findings would be considered as outcome evaluation?

ECONOMIC EVALUATION

Economics in health promotion is concerned with estimating the relative value of a programme or intervention in relation to its health benefit. It aims to assist policy-makers to set priorities in the longer term to improve efficiency by converting 'inputs' such as money or labour into 'outputs' such as health gain or saving lives. Economic evaluation uses a variety of tools such as cost minimisation analysis, cost effective analysis, cost benefit analysis and cost utility analysis (Drummond et al., 2005). Cost minimisation analysis looks at the cheapest intervention by comparing costs of achieving a given outcome. Cost effective analysis measures the consequences of intervention measured often in years gained or lives saved. Cost benefit analysis uses monetary terms and is centred on how much money is spent or saved. Cost utility analysis is interested in both quality and quantity of life and health outcomes. QALY (quality adjusted life year) is a commonly used measure of health benefit in economic evaluation particularly cost utility analysis. For a summary of these methods see Figure 8.5.

 In health promotion there is often a trade-off between efficiency (costs and benefits) and equal access to health benefits. It is argued for example that before new vaccines are incorporated into the WHO and *UNICEF* supported Extended Programme of Immunisation (EPI) developing countries should be increasing their coverage of existing vaccines. The coverage rate varies between 50 and 80% so large numbers of the population are already not benefiting from the programme. Spending therefore on new vaccines will increase this inequality (WHO, 2010).

Analysis type	Analysis methods
Cost minimisation	• Compares costs of interventions to achieve the same outcome • Often used in pharmacology to compare drugs, i.e. generic vs non-generic
Cost effectiveness	• Measures outcomes of health interventions in terms of units, e.g. years of life gained • Does not question rationale for doing the intervention but how much of the intervention should be done
Cost benefit	• Deals in monetary terms, e.g. how much have we saved? • Asks whether the benefits outweigh the costs • Widely used in economic evaluation
Cost utility	• Measures both quality and quantity of health outcomes • States of health are valued in relation to one another • Looks at the cost of the additional years of life and the quality of life • QALY often used as a tool

Figure 8.5   Economic cost analysis types

PARTICIPATORY EVALUATION

Participatory evaluation is the primary feature of community health-based programmes. It takes a pluralistic approach with the aim that individuals within the community are not only benefiting from the programme but also participating in its planning and implementation. Participatory evaluation recognises that when assessing the efficacy of an intervention, each individual or group will have a different perspective. All health promotion programmes will have a number of stakeholders whose influence and power on the outcomes of the programme will be unequal. Participatory evaluation seeks to challenge the idea that everyone wants the same things and that there is a common set of values for a programme.

Speaking at a conference in Japan to discuss the health programme and future for Fukushima Prefecture following the devastating tsunami, Kamiya (2012) emphasised the importance of direct involvement of residents, experts in the local area, authorities managing the situation and public health representatives in the planning and decision-making for the future. He drew on the radiological protection strategies developed in Belarus following the Chernobyl incident where resident participation has shaped the management of the long-term effects of the contamination (Lochard, 2004).

ACTIVITY 8.5
Participatory involvement

Re-read the section on participatory evaluation.

1 If you were a resident in the Fukushima Prefecture what direct involvement might you want to see?
2 How might this be achieved?

EXPERIMENTAL DESIGN EVALUATION

Experimental evaluation in health generally compares the success of an intervention by making comparisons with those who have been exposed to an intervention with those who have not. It can also measure the before-and-after effects of a programme and tends to report on specific health outcomes. The application of this type of evaluation involves establishing 'variables' which can be defined as characteristics such as age or gender that may influence any result. Randomised control trials (RCTs) are seen as the most reliable method. There are two main tenets of an RCT. People are randomly allocated to a study group and there need to be at least two groups for comparison. They are widely used in therapeutic decision-making such as clinical trials to determine the efficacy of a drug regime. Traditionally RCTs are seen as being limited in coping with complex health promotion programmes because they do not measure process outcomes or qualitative data. Conversely those undertaking RCTs do not always value qualitative or 'perceived' less rigorous testing. This has been refuted by a number of researchers. See Chapter 7 for more on RCTs and evidence.

RELIABILITY AND VALIDITY

Research outcomes are usually measured in terms of their reliability. Reliability is concerned with achieving consistent results even when the activity is repeated. Health promoters would be unable to develop theories or draw conclusions if reliable tools were not available to them. For example, a programme to promote smoking cessation in Russia where it is deemed a major public health issue may use scare tactic messages to target young women. These messages may be replicated in the Ukraine among a target group matched for age, ethnicity, socioeconomic status, profession and living in an urban environment. The results may show that the scare tactics work in Russia but not in the Ukraine.

Another way of ensuring that findings are credible is through the use of internal and external validity measurement. Internal validity measures the extent to which the results are deemed accurate due to the intervention itself and not other factors. In other words the right things were measured. External validity is concerned with how the results can be extrapolated for wider use. Thorogood and Coombes (2010) postulate that there will always be tension between external and internal validity. Internal validity is seen as requiring rigorous experimental research methods often using gold standard quantitative methods such as RCTs. Evaluation will tend to focus on impact and outcomes. Conversely, external validity will use a host of methods both qualitative and quantitative and will use more formative and process evaluation. For an example of external validity see Case Study 8.3.

Case Study 8.3

Evaluation of video-based decision aid

Albrecht et al. (2011) examined how a German audience appraised an American video-based decision aid on early stage breast cancer.

Methods used were:

- A German synchronised voice-over version of the decision aid was shown to focus groups comprising patients, health care providers and health care experts. An individual questionnaire was used together with a moderated group discussion. Research questions included an appraisal of the decision aid and its adaptation for use in Germany.

- Positive findings suggested the majority of health experts (100%), patients (86%) and health care providers (71%) thought the decision aid was good or very good. There were also a number of negative findings. The negative findings focused on the aid being too American, with the setting and environment being too different and the German voice-over version was seen as negative. They concluded that despite a high level of interest and positive appraisal of the decision aid the study suggests that it cannot just be translated and used in another country.

EVALUATING INTERVENTIONS USING THEORETICAL MODELS OF COMMUNICATION

The examples in this section demonstrate how theoretical models can be used to evaluate health communication. Chapter 1 explores theoretical models of communication and their application to health promotion practice. Theoretical models help to frame the planning and evaluation process but in practice they are often modified or used with other models. This helps to avoid the pitfalls of applying a rigid framework to a complex area of predicting human behaviour and experience. Most health communication models are based on behaviours that are health related or health seeking. They identify variables and specify how these work to achieve an outcome. For example, accessing health care. The model together with the variables such as age, gender and equality will depend on the target population and what appeals to them (Witte, 2007).

Theory and evaluation

Twomby et al. (2008) undertook an intervention using the theory of planned behaviour (TPB), which focuses on the theory that beliefs and knowledge in turn influence intentions and behaviour (see Chapter 1 for an explanation of this model).

The study involved the evaluation of a science curriculum which covered drugs of abuse. School-based health programmes are perceived to be effective but health programmes are often a low priority within the school curriculum. It was decided to introduce drug education into the science curriculum using an interactive multi-media programme. The aims of the programme were to find out:

- How did the knowledge of drugs change pre- and post-test?
- What is the effect of multi-media on knowledge change?
- To what extent did group assignment relate to change in knowledge?
- How do factors such as protective attitudes towards drugs change with knowledge?
- What is the statistical effect when variables such as gender and race are included?

(Continued)

Case Study 8.4

(Continued)

Eight schools participated. Four schools undertook the interactive multi-media curriculum (experimental group); four schools undertook the traditional science programme with health education as a separate subject (control group).
Evaluation methods included:

- A multiple choice test pre- and post-intervention.
- An attitude survey on how likely negative health, social, academic and legal outcomes were attributed to drug abuse.

The experimental group using the multi-media science resources demonstrated a significant change in knowledge and attitudes to drug abuse while the control group demonstrated little change.

The transtheoretical model (TTM) is used widely in health communication. Its advantage is its relative simplicity. It involves six stages whereby the individual goes through stages of precontemplation, contemplation, preparation, action, maintenance and maybe relapse (see Chapter 1). Stephenson and Stephenson (2011) used the TTM alongside the health belief model (HBM) to develop a training programme to prevent hearing loss among carpenters. A survey tool was developed to test the attitudes, beliefs and social norms related to hearing protection use and behavioural intentions following completion of the training. Bleakley et al. (2011) used the integrative model of behavioural prediction (this includes the health belief model, social cognitive theory and the theory of reasoned action; see Fishbein and Capella, 2006) to determine how exposure to sexual media content influences sexual behaviour in adolescents. The research demonstrated that the intention to engage in sexual intercourse was affected by attitude, normative pressure and self-efficacy. Exposure to sexual media content, however, only affects normative beliefs. Case Study 8.4 is an example of theory in evaluation.

WHAT TO MEASURE IN EVALUATION

The questions how do we know if the intervention was successful and how will we measure the success are achieved by initially having clear objectives and indicators for success. This is why it is important to decide on the evaluation process at the planning stage of the intervention. Objectives often ask these questions. Who is the audience that the intervention is aimed at? What change is needed? How much change and what is the timescale? Indicators for success should be designed specifically to measure progress linked to the objective. The indicators should also be valid and accessible to the target population. They should be clear about what is being measured and how the information will be collected.

Methods used in evaluation will vary depending on the type of intervention that is undertaken. Having clear objectives and indicators will assist the evaluator in

Objective	Possible evaluation method
To increase knowledge e.g. How HIV spreads	Pre- and post-test questionnaire, observation in practice, using experimental and control groups
To change behaviour e.g. correct insulin injecting procedures	Record number of clients undertaking behaviour
To change attitude and values e.g. breast milk is best for babies	Focus groups, one-to-one interviews
To establish health-promoting environments e.g. community gardens, cycle lanes	Measure cycling flows and visits to gardens
To enhance decision-making skills e.g. healthy food choices	Observe a demonstration in a group or individually
To change policy e.g. outdoor non-smoking area	Record legislative changes
To raise health awareness e.g. exercise programmes	Record how many people took leaflets or attended the sessions
To improve health status e.g. a reduction in blood pressure	Keep records of health indicators

Figure 8.6 Examples of evaluation methods matched to objectives

their choice of data gathering. There should also be a process by which unforeseen outcomes are recorded. Process evaluation methods will often be appropriate in those instances, for example, if an intervention is seen to be failing because there has been a bus strike and clients cannot attend the focus groups.

Figure 8.6 gives examples of the type of objective for a programme and the evaluation method that could be used.

It is important that standards can be applied to the evaluation of health communication to avoid the pitfalls associated with poorly planned interventions such as poor use of resources and lack of credible evidence to add to the overall knowledge base. The Healthy People 2020 project (US Office of Disease Prevention and Health Promotion, 2010) cites the following standards for educational evaluation to be used in health promotion programmes. They are:

- *Utility* (Is it useful?)
- *Feasibility* (Does it make sense?)
- *Propriety* (Is it ethical?)
- *Accuracy* (Are the findings correct?)

Figure 8.7 covers the key elements required in assessing whether health communication has been effective.

Accuracy	Is the content valid? Are there any factual errors?
Availability	Is the content delivery or venue accessible?
Balance	Does the content show the risks and benefits?
Consistency	Is the content consistent over time?
Cultural competence	Does the design account for variables such as ethnicity, race and language?
Evidence base	Has the relevant evidence undergone analysis and review to formulate practice guidelines?
Reach	Does the information reach the target population?
Reliability	Are sources credible and up to date?
Repetition	Is delivery or access to information continued or repeated to reinforce impact?
Timeliness	Is content available or provided when the audience is most in need or susceptible to it?
Understanding	Is the reading language or format appropriate?

Figure 8.7   Suggestions for the evaluation of effective health communication, adapted from Healthy People 2020 (US Office of Disease Prevention and Health Promotion, 2000)

ACTIVITY 8.6
Ways to evaluate health communication

A campaign to promote the uptake of sport in the over-fifties age group in a rural area was undertaken under the auspices of the London Olympics' aim to get more people participating in sport. Four leisure centres took part in the campaign with support from Sport for England and two local authorities. Using the headings in Figure 8.7. How would you evaluate this campaign?

EVALUATION OF MASS COMMUNICATION

The relationship between health communication and mass media is one that has both positive and negative characteristics. Health-related articles appear in newspapers, on radio and television and on the Internet daily. They can be informative or misleading. They can also be helpful in dissemination of information in health crises such as pandemic influenza and they can militate against the success of campaigns through conflicts of self interest between health care lobbies (Guida, 2010). The strengths of mass media lie in their ability to get messages out to a wide audience and to get simple public health issues on to the agenda. A WHO and UNICEF campaign to encourage the take up of zinc supplementation as part of the treatment for diarrhoea in children under five years in Nepal was assisted by a mass communication strategy. The findings showed that behaviour towards the use of zinc was positively associated with the recall of information via the mass media programme (Wang et al., 2011). Mass communication rarely works on its own and does not deal well with complex messages (see Chapter 4). It is also less useful in teaching skills and changing attitudes and behaviours (Thorogood and Coombes, 2010). It can be difficult to evaluate the effects of mass communication predominately because the main forms of mass media utilise one message for a mass audience. Two possible methods are monitoring and media analysis.

MONITORING CAMPAIGNS

Monitoring involves the systematic collection of information that will help to answer questions about the intervention or programme. It tracks the implementation process and observes the progress of the programme against time, resources and impact. It is used in conjunction with evaluation but is limited in its scope. It tends to measure timings and frequencies of interventions and differs in the types of questions it asks. Monitoring a programme will involve first, keeping records of the nature of the participants; second, the interventions that they receive; and third, tracking the progress towards programme objectives (Fertman and Allensworth, 2010). The information is collected using a database, many of which can be located through library sources or on the Internet.

The steps involved in collecting data would include identifying areas where feedback is required and developing a reporting pro forma. The Charities Evaluation Service (2012) suggests a number of possible ways to ensure effective monitoring:

- Keep stakeholders fully informed. This prompts useful questions about activities and prompts corrective action.
- Select key indicators and collect data regularly to track progress.
- Distinguish between new and repeat users by categories to ensure accuracy
- Break down data by category, e.g. gender, age, ethnicity. Use validated tools for this purpose, e.g. those used by the Equality and Human Rights Commission in England.
- Be mindful of the Data Protection Act. Ensure confidentiality, make sure the data are used for their intended purpose and keep stakeholders informed of what is being held.

When undertaking monitoring of media campaigns it is important that the monitoring process is clear at the outset. Findings can be very powerful if undertaken on a large scale. The Global Media Monitoring Project (GMMP, 2010) focuses on measuring the representation of women in the media. The tool used is divided up into seven areas namely: politics and government; economy, science and health; social and legal; crime and violence; celebrity, arts and media; sports; and girl-child. This project, which has been running since 1995, demonstrates that there is poor representation of women in the media and it is not improving. The publication 'Who makes the news?' (GMMP, 2010) showed that only 24% of those heard or read about in radio, television, print and online are female. In the area of science and health 32% are female. These findings have far-reaching implications for empowerment and social exclusion as media dictate women's roles and opportunities in society.

MEDIA ANALYSIS

Health promoters and communicators need to be aware of the machinations of the mass media in order to understand how to present important health messages in an effective way. In order to evaluate how the health messages are being presented through the media, a media analysis can be conducted. The analysis involves locating articles relating to the health messages using agreed search words. The search is restricted to a specific time frame and this would probably relate to the timing of the campaign. The articles are then entered into a date-restricted news database. Commonly used examples are Google News and LexisNexis (Corcoran, 2011). Once the information is collected a set of criteria is applied to measure how the campaign is being presented. Figure 8.8 shows examples of questions.

Question	Example
How do the media frame public attitudes to a health campaign?	What are the elements? Is the language used consistent?
Who are the spokespeople and how are they quoted?	Are they advocates, policy-makers, health experts, celebrities, scientists?
How are they quoted and in what context?	Are they quoted consistently? Is the context appropriate to the campaign?
What is being emphasised? What is being ignored?	Are the key messages being compromised?
Which media are covering or ignoring the issue?	Is the coverage in visual, spoken, written or Internet-based media?
Are there seasonal differences in coverage?	Is there less coverage because the weather has changed?
Is it front page news or low profile?	Is the message losing its impact?

Figure 8.8   Key questions for media analysis, adapted from Gould (2004)

EVALUATING ONLINE CAMPAIGNS

The use of the Internet in health campaigns is becoming increasingly popular. Health websites have been available for many years and are a popular form of health information. As the Internet population grows exponentially the use of web-based health advice will be the most popular medium. Evaluating e-based programmes is always difficult and for the users of the sites the major concerns lie around the validity of the information provided. The National Cancer Institute in the USA provided a guide on questions to ask when accessing information about cancer on the Internet (National Cancer Institute, 2010). The questions include: Who manages the information? Who funds the project? And what is the original source of information?

Developing areas in health promotion concern the harnessing of social media sites to improve communication in health campaigns. Sites such as Facebook, Twitter and MySpace all have huge potential for health communication. The FaceSpace project is a sexual health promotion intervention which uses social networking sites. This approach allows the sharing of information and interactive activities. The challenge for health promoters is to develop appropriate evaluation tools to explore the health outcomes from this approach. O'Grady et al. (2009) propose a framework which incorporates technologies that facilitate collaboration among users in a traditional or novel way. They describe these technologies as collaborative, adaptive and interactive. The proposal includes formative, process and outcome evaluation using five indicators, namely:

- *People:* Those who use or have developed the site.
- *Content:* Including text, images and multimedia.
- *Technology:* Underlying technology to create and run the site.
- *Computer-mediated interaction:* Assessment of user interaction with and via the interface.
- *Health systems integration:* The integration of the technology into the wider health system.

The use of mobile devices is also changing the face of health communication. Text4Baby (2012) is a free mobile health information service to improve maternal and child health in America. Expectant mothers can sign up and receive advice via their mobile phones. The first evaluation as part of ongoing research demonstrated that there was a high level of satisfaction with the service particularly with the Spanish-speaking version (Text4Baby, 2010).

DISSEMINATION OF RESULTS

Dissemination of results is the final stage in the evaluation cycle. It is essential that outcomes are shared with all the participants, policy-makers and the wider public. It is the right of all stakeholders to have access to the knowledge and potential benefits of the programme. Coombes (2010) observes that often dissemination is focused on the decision makers rather than the participants and this is ethically unsound. Case Study 8.5 demonstrates the importance of dissemination and feedback to participants.

The National Child Measurement Programme

The National Child Measurement Programme was launched against the background of increasing child obesity. Data are collected on height and weight of all children aged between 4 and 11 in all primary schools in England. In order to raise awareness of the importance of healthy weight and to engage families in healthy lifestyle issues, the Primary Care Trusts (PCTs) have provided feedback to parents on their child's height and weight in the form of a letter and leaflet. A small-scale study in four PCTs was undertaken. The two aims of the study were to explore the impact of parents receiving routine feedback and to learn from this experience. The majority of parents agreed with the results and found the information helpful. Parents of the overweight children were less satisfied and some parents reacted to the harsh language used. Nearly a third of the parents stated that they would take action although later evidence demonstrated that little action had been taken (see Mooney et al., 2010).

Dissemination helps to ensure that the findings are embedded in future policies and health programmes and also assists in the building of a credible evidence base. The process of dissemination needs to be systematic and well planned and will require resources. It is important that there is a strategy for demonstrating the relevance of the findings for future practice and to think about whether a recommendation for adopting the findings is included in the dissemination process if appropriate. There are barriers to effective dissemination and these include:

- There may be competing professional priorities in an organisation or among stakeholders.
- The language used may not be understood by all.
- The less empowered may not get access to information due to not receiving information in an appropriate form or lack of access.
- There may be technical barriers such as difficulty using the Internet.
- The choice of methods may be inappropriate.

ACTIVITY 8.7
Bullying among young teenagers

You are planning to disseminate information on a recent programme to tackle bullying in a large comprehensive school in a large city. The main findings show a decrease in reported bullying among boys in years 7 and 8 but no change in reporting in girls of the same age.

1   How will you disseminate these findings and to whom?
2   What barriers could you encounter?

CONCLUSION

Evaluation is an essential part of health communication practice. Methods employed in evaluating a programme or interventions are numerous and need to be employed to reflect the complexity of most health communication. Tried and tested models of formative, process, impact and outcome evaluation form the bedrock of assessment. New models however are required to find effective ways of evaluating online health promotion as this becomes a more common approach. Evaluation should be planned at the start of a programme and continued throughout and beyond. Findings should be disseminated to all stakeholders regardless of their perceived status. Good quality evaluation will add to the body of evidence to improve health outcomes.

Summary

- This chapter has examined the role and importance of evaluation in health communication.
- Theoretical models of evaluation have been explored including the formative, process, impact and outcome model. Other models explored are economic and participatory evaluation, and use of theoretical models in relation to evaluation are discussed.
- The chapter highlights aspects of media evaluation including evaluation of online programmes using social networking sites, monitoring and media analysis.
- Dissemination of findings and the rationale for engagement in this process have been discussed.

ADDITIONAL READING

There is a chapter on designated practical evaluation in Corcoran N (2011) *Working on Health Communication*. Sage, London.

A good overall textbook centred on evaluation is Thorogood M and Coombes Y (2010) (eds) *Evaluating Health Promotion: Practice and methods*, 3rd edition. Oxford University Press, Oxford.

9

BRIDGING THEORY AND PRACTICE – TEN DIFFERENT HEALTH PROMOTION CAMPAIGNS

NOVA CORCORAN

Communicating Health: Strategies for health promotion has explored eight areas of communication in health promotion and health education practice. Now readers should be in a position to commence the design of communication strategies, to utilise methods and to undertake practice around communication design. This book concludes with 10 different health promotion related campaigns to enable health practitioners to see models of good work in practice.

This section is designed to encourage exploration of the 10 campaigns that have used a variety of strategies and methods to achieve their goals. They include many of the elements discussed in this textbook and embody the philosophy of promoting health in a number of ways, bringing together a variety of practitioners and ideas to achieve their aims. This is not a definitive list of health promotion campaigns, but is designed to encourage the reader to explore what works, and gain ideas and insights to inform their own practice. Although there are other campaigns that could have been chosen, these were selected because they are recent, cover a variety of audiences, topics and goals, and are accessible to the reader via the Internet. Health practitioners are encouraged to spend time looking at these campaigns via the websites provided to gain a final overview of how the theoretical concepts of this textbook are linked to practice.

1   THE USE OF THEORY IN A CAMPAIGN: FOOD DUDES

Food Dudes appeals to young children from 4 to 11 years old, and involves a set of steps revolving around a reward system, a DVD adventure (starring the Food Dudes) and repeated tasting of foods which has been shown to increase intake of fruit and vegetables. It is aimed at primary school children to increase fruit and vegetable intake. The main philosophy is that rewards and positive role models help to increase consumption. See the main campaign website for resources and other campaign information at www.fooddudes.co.uk/.

2   THE USE OF MULTI-MEDIA STRATEGIES IN HEALTH PROMOTION: THINK ROAD SAFETY

The Department for Transport (DfT) focuses on a range of driving-related areas in its campaign Think! including drink-driving, drug-driving, motorbikes, road safety, speeding and fatigue. It contains a range of materials including wider media for use in schools or youth groups and education resources on road crossing. Road safety messages are also disseminated at the roadside, for example, using the rear tailgates of trucks with messages such as 'Don't drive tired'. The website contains a range of resources including a game which aims to illustrate the difficulty of driving while doing two things at once (talking on your mobile phone and driving). See this campaign at http://think.direct.gov.uk/.

3   A CAMPAIGN THAT FRAMES A HEALTH ISSUE DIFFERENTLY: 'SAVE THE CRABS AND EAT 'EM'

This campaign aims to discourage the use of fertilisers in the Chesapeake Bay area at certain times of the year as the run-off pollutes the water where the seafood lives. This campaign aimed to reduce fertiliser use by focusing on the Chesapeake blue crabs and seafood that is consumed in the bay. The audience were predominately urban, and the campaign designers wanted to overcome message fatigue from previous bay-orientated campaigns by promoting a connection with the bay area. The campaign message was framed not as an environmental appeal, but as a way to ensure the continued availability of Chesapeake Bay seafood. See the posters, videos and other information at www.chesapeakeclub.org/media.shtml and http://thensmc.com/resources/showcase/save-the-crabs.

4   A CAMPAIGN THAT AIMS TO TEACH A SKILL: 'HARD AND FAST'

The British Heart Foundation (BHF, 2012) use a television advert featuring ex-football player and actor Vinnie Jones who performs hands only CPR while giving instructions to his audience The main message is 'Hands only CPR – hard and fast'. You can also use a downloadable iPhone/android app to practise hands only CPR. The website also contains answers to frequently asked questions and social media links (i.e. a blog and Twitter feed). See the campaign at www.bhf.org.uk/heart-health/life-saving-skills/hands-only-cpr.aspx.

5   A CAMPAIGN BASED ON AN IDENTIFIED KNOWLEDGE GAP: CHLAMYDIA WORTH TALKING ABOUT

Research suggests that fostering a culture that frames sexual behaviour among young people as a normal part of their development is better for sexual health promotion. The chlamydia strand of the NHS sexual health campaign Sex Worth Talking About highlights the potential infertility that untreated chlamydia cases can cause. It also focuses on the fact that chlamydia is spreading, is symptomless, but is easy and painless to diagnose and treat. You can view the chlamydia worth talking about television advert at www.nhs.uk/Video/Pages/chlamydia-worth-talking-about.aspx. Campaign resources are available at www.nhs.uk/sexualhealthprofessional/Pages/campaign-resources.aspx.

6   A CAMPAIGN TO ADVOCATE PUBLIC POLICY CHANGES: ARE WE TAKING THE DIS?

The Disability Rights Commission (2006) is campaigning to change Britain and put disability at the heart of public policy. They propose 10 priorities for change, including increasing disabled people's participation, closing the employment gap, supporting independent living and promoting children's life chances. The Are We Taking the Dis? campaign aims to highlight the inequity and inequalities experienced by those with a disability. 'I earn less than my colleagues just for being deaf', or 'I'm a real fashion victim, I can't get into the shops' are just two of the advertising messages encouraging debates, forums and discussions around disability. You can view the campaign at www.drc.org.uk/disabilitydebate.

7   A SETTINGS-BASED HEALTH PROMOTION CAMPAIGN: BBHOP

The Black Barbershop Health Outreach Program (BBHOP) aims to address health care disparities in African American men. It has been running since 2006 with a focus on diabetes, high blood pressure and prostate cancer. The original aim of the programme was to reach African American men who were at risk for cardiovascular disease. Black-owned barber shops were seen to represent a setting which regularly attracts the target group and provides a location where health education could be disseminated. It focuses on cities across America (38 currently). Volunteers measure blood pressure and screen for diabetes and refer on to medical services as necessary. The primary aim is to screen, educate (through a variety of health education messages and strategies) and refer as required. More recently the initiative has launched a black beautyshop campaign aimed at African American women. You can view this campaign at http://blackbarbershop.org/.

8 A CAMPAIGN THAT AIMS TO CHANGE BEHAVIOUR: WHY LET GOOD TIMES GO BAD

Why Let Good Times Go Bad is a Drinkaware (2011) campaign aimed at encouraging young adults to have a good time while drinking alcohol rather than a bad time. This focuses not on telling the target audience to not drink, but to drink in a safer way. One of the messages, for example, is 'have something to eat to stay on your feet'. A range of campaign materials have been produced including posters with a good/bad split, a video that provides a parody alternative to a popular music video, as well as a mobile app to track drinks. See the video at www.drinkaware. co.uk/campaigns/2011/why-let-good-times-go-bad-2011/katy-perry-video. See all the campaign resources including the phone app and posters at www.drinkaware. co.uk/campaigns/2011/why-let-good-times-go-bad-2011.

9 A CAMPAIGN TO PROVIDE INFORMATION TO A SPECIFIC AUDIENCE: THE MIDDLE AGE SPREAD

In 2010 the Family Planning Association (FPA) ran the first ever national sexual health campaign for people over 50. They centred on the fact that people in their fifties, sixties, seventies and eighties are having sex with new partners. There is increasing growth of STIs in older age groups but condom use may be ignored due to the association of condoms with pregnancy. See the posters and campaign information at www.fpa.org.uk/campaignsandadvocacy/sexualhealthweek/stisandsafersexover50.

10 A CAMPAIGN DESIGNED TO CHANGE LIFESTYLE-RELATED BEHAVIOUR: SWAP IT DON'T STOP IT

The Australian government's healthy lifestyle campaign focuses on 'swapping', for example 'big for small', or 'sitting for moving'. The campaign website gives reasons and ways to swop alongside a 'swap of the day' (e.g. swap your evening dessert for an evening walk), a postcode activity finder and food swap ideas. You can watch the TV adverts at http://swapit.gov.au/resources and view the campaign website and resources at http://swapit.gov.au/.

A similar UK campaign aimed at changing healthy lifestyles is the DH Change4Life campaign, which you can view at www.nhs.uk/Change4Life/Pages/change-for-life.aspx.

ACTIVITY DISCUSSIONS

This section contains discussions from the activities throughout the textbook. They are designed not as definitive answers, but as suggested examples to the activities.

CHAPTER 1

1.1   How are health promotion messages communicated?

1   Traditional sources of communication such as television, radio, magazines, news-papers, Internet, telephone, one-to-one alongside more non-traditional sources such as sign language, symbols, text messages or eye contact.
2   Interpersonal information (one-to-one or group work) or different types of media including mass media (newspapers, magazines, television), print media (leaflets, booklets, posters), electronic media (Internet) and audio visual (radio, video).

1.2   Why not use theory?

1   Time, resources, finance, lack of expertise or difficulty of application to practice.

1.3   The theory of planned behaviour in action

1   Yes, Daniel will probably take the steroids. Look again at Figure 1.5, and follow the format. He has a positive attitude (wants to look good) and a supportive subjective norm (a member of staff with 'muscles' already using steroids). Perceived behavioural control is more difficult; we are not sure if he is ready, willing and can access steroids, but will assume that he can. With regard to strong behavioural intention, all pointers indicate that he will try steroids to look good, resulting in the action of taking the steroids.

1.4   The perceived behavioural control (PBC) model in action

1   At the 'preknowledge' stage you would provide information or resources to move people to the 'knowledge' stage. At the 'knowledge' stage people would need to

gain some knowledge about recycling and the facilities available. At the 'approval' stage people would agree that recycling bins are a good idea, and that recycling rubbish is a positive step. At the 'intention' stage, people would need to intend to recycle, for example, next time they have a collection of glass or paper. At the 'practice' stage people would be actively recycling their glass or paper. Finally, at the 'advocacy' stage they would be encouraging others to do the same.

1.5   How are health promotion messages communicated?

1   A number of variables could be targeted. You could target social norms or perceived behavioural control from the theory of planned behaviour. You could also target perceived susceptibility or severity from the health belief model.
2   What sort of messages would you target at the constructs of this model to promote safer sexual relationships? This depends on the model you chose. One example might be a message that focuses on 'your friends and family would like you to use a condom when you hook up to protect yourself' (social norms), or 'don't be scared to use a condom – you have the power to insist' (perceived behavioural control).

CHAPTER 2

2.1   Differences in health behaviours

1   Different emphasis on preventive behaviours, including screening, and may have different health-related behaviours with regard to issues such as sexual health, safety or physical activity. There may also be differences in lifestyles that impact on health, for example levels of physical activity or dietary differences.
2   Different concerns; for example, females may have concerns around menopause or osteoporosis, in addition there may be family or religious restrictions in terms of exercise and diet. Males may have less concern for their health, or be focused on illness only when it becomes serious. Males and females are at different risks for different diseases in later life, for example men have a higher risk of CHD. In addition certain cancers are more prevalent in men (i.e. prostate cancer) and women (breast or cervical cancer).

2.2   Messages for education levels

1   The Diabetes UK website has less text and more interactive features including images and pictures. The NHS website has more text and is less obvious to navigate. Both sites are very comprehensive but finding the exact information

may prove difficult to those less computer literate. Interactive tools such as those that calculate diabetes risk encourage engagement with the site.

2   Difficulties may arise for those whose levels of English are low as there is much written material on both sites. There may be a personal preference for websites depending on colour, format, ease of navigation and ease of finding information that is being searched for.

2.3   Who is the message designed for?

1   Age: Mid- to older age adults (note the picture) who are at risk of bowel cancer.
2   There is no definite answer here, but as the doctor is male it is possible the rationale was to focus more on males who are at risk.
3   Socioeconomic: all inclusive as little writing means it is accessible to all. Those who are most likely to access a doctor for screening however are the middle and upper socioeconomic groups.
4   Education: little writing, few complex instructions and accessible to all groups.
5   Ethnicity: The doctor shown is Asian, which would suggest this particular poster is aimed at Asian groups, or those living in areas with a reasonable prevalence of Asian doctors such as large cities.
6   There are differences in target group, i.e. age, the focus of the message and the type of images use (cartoon compared to photo). There are similarities in terms of the simplicity of the message and the education/socioeconomic class being less important to the overall message.

2.4   Psychological variables and MMR

Your answer will vary depending on whether you have read any of the research around the vaccine, if you have read any of the stories in the media, what your friends and family think including parents and siblings. Your answer may also be based on knowing someone who has had the vaccine safely and your familiarities with autism and what it is. These variables will form your attitudes to the MMR and will impact on a decision to vaccinate a child.

2.5   Attitudes and complexity

1   A positive attitude to bowel cancer screening as a person has known someone else who has had the screening, read a leaflet or watched a documentary on bowel cancer.
2   A negative attitude to bowel cancer screening as a person may think it is invasive, that they are not at risk, that it is something that happens to other people.

3   A positive attitude to HIV tests as a person has known other people who have been tested, they have been tested in the past and think that it is a good idea in terms of letting a partner know they are HIV free.
4   A negative attitude to HIV testing as a person may consider it a personal issue, be worried about being tested positive, be concerned about insurance or employment, think that HIV is a 'curse' or that they will be stigmatised.

2.6   Beliefs and tobacco

1   A wide range of reasons which could include; 'it makes me look cool, sexy, good looking, older, thinner, wiser, sophisticated or grown up'. 'It keeps my weight down', 'it's good for me', 'it helps my lungs', 'my doctor said it is good for me', 'it helps me relax'.
2   You could target any of these beliefs. For example with teenagers messages for those who believe it makes them look older could focus on wrinkles or poor skin. Messages for those who believe it makes them look 'cool' could focus on smelly clothes or bad breath.

2.7   Designing messages to target attitudes

1   This answer will depend on your target group. An example might be 16-year-old black African girls who are leaving school with few qualifications (lower education levels).
2   Messages that could be developed to target this group might centre around chlamydia being invisible and serious. In terms of personal relevance it could look at promoting condom use not just for contraceptive effect but for chlamydia prevention as well. Messages would perhaps focus on African girls in workplaces such as shops or beauty salons as places of work after leaving school or could be disseminated in this way.

CHAPTER 3

3.1   Cultural identity

1   This is subjective and may centre on your own religious beliefs, behaviours or traditions, among other factors.
2   Examples include: different beliefs than others, different attitudes, judgemental or discriminatory practices or inability to communicate in a different language.
3   Embrace diversity and difference, consider non-traditional ways of communicating or ensure adequate translation services are available.

3.2   Barriers to health

1   Location of services, language barriers, cultural differences, late presentation of signs/symptoms, accessibility of services, difficulties in translating materials, fear of the unknown and lack of experience accessing Western health services.
2   Examples include: provide additional information resources (e.g. leaflets or booklets), encourage talk between staff/patients and patient/patient, or allow time for questions in consultations and ensure the target group is aware of these issues. Images need to be culturally relevant and as a basic requirement information provision should be in a range of formats and languages.

3.3   Challenging the present

1   Aside from the last example (outcomes of care), all of these involve contact between the user of a service and the provider of a service – either a mental health-related service or other authority (e.g. police).
2   Projects could include: advocacy workers in these settings to encourage good communication, campaigns to reduce stigma of mental illness, promoting understanding of different cultural beliefs around mental illness and mental health in the wider community, providing support for those identified as at risk, either emotional or resource based.

3.4   Disability campaigns

1   Messages focus around rights and inclusion in health services. Methods include multi-media strategies not dissimilar to other campaigns.
2   The main aims focus around reducing hate crime through advocacy and awareness, and enabling access to screening services through increasing knowledge and awareness.
3   This depends on your personal opinion, but advocacy and awareness raising are helpful as a starting point but may not always translate into action especially when others are involved in the health care process who may know about these campaigns, e.g. health care workers.
4   Further advocacy, for example a focus on other areas such as health care workers might be helpful as a two-part strategy. Other forms of multiple media might be helpful, such as information technology.

3.5   'Stop smoking' materials for those over 70

1   A large font would be preferable on written material, and use of audio materials should be considered. Use of an appropriate planning, implementation and

evaluation framework should be used alongside the appropriate theoretical model.

2 No. Materials in this setting should use a combination of media.

3.6 'Healthy heart' programme design

1 Encourage health professionals to make a referral to the class, telephone individuals, provide refreshments, offer one-to-one sessions alongside the group classes.
2 Making friends, appearance related or getting out of the house.
3 Website, telephone or mobile technology-based support.

3.7 National Service Framework demonstrated outcomes

Example: Flu immunisation

1 A well-planned advertising campaign, letters from GP practices to all those at risk, provision of drop-in clinics (no appointments) to increase uptake.
2 Message design would focus on 'keeping well' in the winter, or keeping fit in the winter, the fact that it is easy to protect oneself, and free.

3.8 Older people and sexual health

1 This could be an extension of other sexual health campaigns, or be included in older people focused websites such as Age UK. See Chapter 9 for the example of the middle age spread campaign. Health care professionals will need to consider that sexual health for older people is still a real issue and that STIs may still be prevalent in an older age group.
2 Freedom of communication and travel may promote sexual relationships, and changes to family structure, i.e. divorce and re-marriages in later life, may also promote STIs. The promotion of condoms for prevention of pregnancy in young people may mean that older people are missed out of sexual health focused campaigns in terms of STIs and condom use.

CHAPTER 4

4.1 Different media sources

1 1 and 2 You could use a range of different media sources. Here are two examples. Leaflets or posters could use images and slogans to focus on promoting the taste of healthier food such as the sweetness of soft fruit. You could use television

slots to promote how quickly and easily you could cook or prepare vegetables, e.g. a mini cooking programme.

4.2   Mass media and tobacco

1   The advantages of using media include widespread publicity, agenda setting, reaches the whole population, counteracts the pro-smoking lobby, opportunistic, the message that tobacco is a major public health issue. There is limited evidence that mass media are effective using these examples, and are not suitable for all groups; it could give mixed messages, and will not appeal to and reach all groups.
2   One-to-one, skills-based group work, early-school-based education (primary), social marketing strategies may be effective and lobbying the pro-tobacco groups for change (see www.ash.org.uk for more information on lobbying).

4.3   Suitability of methods for mass media

1   Remember that the media cannot teach skills or change strong attitudes. There is a possibility that (a) and (b) could be achieved through mass media.
2   (a) Raising awareness could be achieved via mass media publicity materials. (b) As with (a), mass media could use publicity to advertise a new telephone service. (c) Mass media could provide awareness of a service, but cannot directly increase rates of those screened. (d) Mass media cannot provide skills. (e) Mass media cannot change strong attitudes, but may influence these. Alternative methods include skills-based work and interactive resources that allow active learning.

4.4   A sensible drinking campaign message

1   Sensible drinking words or phrases might include: responsibility, stopping at too much, saying 'no'. Words for those in the 18–25 age group can include: young adults, youth or students. Motivations to 'drink sensibly' can include: unwanted pregnancy, accidents, appearance, not being sick, embarrassment, morning after.
2   An example could be: 'students', 'knowing your limit', 'unwanted pregnancy'.
3   A slogan based on the premise of sticking to a limit, and not experiencing unwanted pregnancy, or emergency contraception, could be 'Remember the night before and forget the morning after'.

4.5   Audience segmentation

1   Groups can include secondary school children, those in a workplace, church-goers, youth groups or young parents.
2   An example setting is a workplace. The group can be split into male/female, older and younger age ranges, those who manage their diabetes themselves,

those who rely on others to manage their diabetes, those who partly manage their diabetes, and those who do not manage their diabetes. These could further be split into those who could manage or could best manage their diabetes through, diet, physical activity, weight control, insulin and so on.

4.6   The four Ps

1   Product: breastfeeding (the practice of this). Price: this can be actual costs positive and negative (i.e. breast milk is free) or perceived costs, embarrassment, perception that it is healthy, reliance on family members so formula feeding its seen as easier, and so on. Place: Location of breastfeeding with very small babies is generally the hospital followed by the home. After this it could then be in any community location, e.g. cafes, library, playgroups. Promotion: want to look at increasing breastfeeding rates so this will be the methods used to promote it – one-to-one support, breastfeeding cafes, breastfeeding-friendly initiatives, etc. Positioning: a message in the location where breastfeeding might take place, e.g. stickers on cafe doors or windows that appeal to the proposed target group.

4.7   Media advocacy

1   Tobacco companies, fast-food manufacturers, non-fair-trade companies or large manufacturers who have lax working or employment laws.
2   An example is tobacco: you can draw attention to the risks of smoking, use case studies to highlight the 'people's' angle, find statistical evidence, use local groups and coalitions or protest and lobby local MPs or local organisations.

4.8   Fear appeals

1   Risks include: loss of memory, inability to function normally, physical or sexual assault and black-outs.
2   Messages can include: keep your drink with you at all times, only accept drinks from people you know, or do not accept drinks you are unsure about or that taste unusual.

CHAPTER 5

5.1   How could IT be used to . . . ?

1   Mobile phones, Internet quizzes, email or touchscreens.
2   Email, Internet, chat rooms, interactive software (e.g. CD-ROMs) or computer games.

5.2   Interactive websites

1   A variety of government, organisational and commercial websites.
2   Websites can contain interactive resources such as alcohol unit calculators, smoking calculators, BMI calculators, diaries, chat rooms, games, activities and quizzes as well as links to blogs, and social media such as Twitter and Facebook.

5.3   SMS messaging services

1   Sexual health messages; some test results; simple information such as appointment reminders; short motivating messages (mental health or physical activity).
2   Complex information; behaviour change information; anything regarded as unwanted information.

5.4   Designing a website

1   Health and hygiene, employment and benefit advice, sources of advice, maintaining positive mental health or information around risky behaviours.
2   As target groups are mixed and it is difficult to identify one single type of user, information should be simple, straightforward and jargon-free, easy to read and navigate, and available in different languages.
3   Accessibility, stigma from the general public, comprehension of information, low literacy levels, poor computer skills.

5.5   Tailoring messages

1   Precontemplation: general information-giving, with advice number if help needed in the future. Contemplation: appealing to current motivations, for example, losing weight before a holiday or big event. Readiness: how to achieve goals, for example, which trainers to buy, which gym class to choose or which nights of the week for walking. Action: advice on keeping going with exercise, tips for low motivation and positive reinforcement of messages. Maintenance: positive reinforcement.

5.6   Health belief model barriers on a website

1   These include cost, habit, taste, price, access, culture, not knowing how to cook, time or children not liking healthy foods.
2   Messages could centre on 'easy' cooking, low prices, sauces and dressings to add variety and taste, and child-friendly meals.

5.7   The seven-step checklist for a website design

An example of website design for this group includes:

1 Interactive media sources such as those in question 5, fact pages, story pages in a magazine format and other ways of presenting information that will appeal to the group.
2 Someone who embodies positive body image and who is of female average size. A health professional may be helpful to answer readers' emails.
3 Ones that embody feeling good about oneself.
4 Colourful, informative and encouraging 'sharing' of information.
5 Quizzes, a chat room or a 'reader's email corner'.
6 Enable anonymous emails.
7 Anywhere where this age group might be found, including university, workplaces, women's groups or other organisations.

CHAPTER 6

6.1   Types of settings for different target groups

Example target group: Primary school children, 5–11 years.

1 Schools, after-school clubs, activity clubs, local community.
2 Mixed or competing messages, parental control, different aims of teachers or the school's governing bodies.

6.2   Fitting activities to settings-based models

1 Organic.
2 Vehicle.
3 Active.
4 Comprehensive.
5 Passive.

6.3   Locations of settings

1 Examples include: Educational: schools, higher education, universities or pre-schools. Health care: primary care, hospitals, dentists, NHS walk-in centres, pharmacists. Social: supermarkets, pubs or workplaces, cinemas, shopping centres.

2   Those settings most widely used include: schools, hospitals, neighbourhoods, workplaces. These are likely to have a bigger reach than some of the smaller settings like barbers or beauty salons.

6.4   Overcoming disadvantages of settings

1   Manpower could involve community or voluntary groups; resources could make use of the wider community and its facilities. Reaching excluded groups will entail choosing different settings, and to include environmental and social aspects, a holistic notion of health will need to be embodied in the whole programme.

6.5   Designing messages for a religious organisation

1   1 and 2 Any religious group could be chosen. Resources can include leaflets or posters with spiritual messages, biblical quotes on materials to encourage healthy behaviours, a prize quiz about aspects of health, competitions, a new website, SMS text messages or other interactive resources.

6.6   Designing a healthy university campaign

You could focus on an issue like healthy food and organise events in the canteen or student union which could include fruit and vegetable taster sessions, information stalls and interactive activities such as cooking demonstrations. These could also be done in halls of residence. Use appropriate-age messages with a catchy theme, show 'student-style' foods, for example pasta or pulses, promote ways to eat more healthily on small budgets. Campaigns could roll through the academic calendar and be integrated into different subjects, for example catering could look at healthy eating menu options, art and design could consider promotion of foods, geography or sociology could look at food choices, transportation of foods and global food issues, and so on.

6.7   Using barbers or beauty salons

Example: Barbers

1   Sexual health, CHD risk, diabetes, prostate cancer, testicular cancer and other areas of high risk.
2   Poor evidence base, so the target group will need to be in close consultation with the project. Access might be difficult and the setting will need to provide a range of opening hours. Limited resources or staff will mean that involving the wider community is essential.

6.8　Settings and convenience stores

1　Tasting stands, promotional fruit or vegetable of the day, traffic light systems of fruit and vegetables, cooking ideas or demonstrations, promotional offers, e.g. 3 for 2.
2　Free take home menus or cooking equipment, collection of vouchers or money off schemes for future purchases, involvement of the main purchaser of food and those who influence the buyer, such as their children.

CHAPTER 7

7.1　Evidence-based practice rationale

1　Evidence embodies the ideals of good practice, it ensures inclusivity and that no-one is excluded or discriminated against. It enables structured working, ensures cooperation, you can help predict any unplanned effects or additional resources and minimise risk of failures.

7.2　What evidence do you use?

1　Community-based work might use 2, 3 and 4. Clinical practice is most likely to use 1 and 2. Students in subjects such as research methods will probably examine the upper of these levels, health policy or local planning might use the lower levels.

7.3　Planning with evidence

1　You could undertake a small pilot study using the council solution (community police officers). You could set up a project that expands on existing projects, for example include 'youths' in this. You could also approach the 'youths' and see what they might want.
2　You should examine other projects in similar neighbourhoods that aim to reduce crime, for example New Deal for Community (NDC) projects or Healthy Cities projects.

7.4　NICE evidence base

1　Their website contains a variety of policy documentation, best practice, evidence-based briefings and other guidelines for good practice. This includes public health guidance on behaviour change, sexual health, accidents, alcohol, tobacco and diabetes.

7.5   Grey literature

1   You could use health impact assessments (HIAs), needs assessments, community profiles, annual reports, minutes of meetings, informal and formal local project reports.
2   You may have been involved in compiling any of these, alongside your more formal work.

7.6   Including developing countries

1   Problems can include: difficulties in representing those with little power; may not be able to reach all of those who should be represented; resource and financial implications; and poor or corrupt management.
2   Suggestions include: start small; try to maintain a base of local projects that can be accessed at national and international level; encourage project leaders to report findings and record these; hold conferences 'on site' rather than in high-class locations; and delegate time and space to listening to others.

7.7   Applicability and transferability

1   Applicability criteria indicate:

- There are few potential barriers.
- The group have expressed an interest so there may be only minor problems in acceptance.
- Contents can be tailored to the new sample; ethnicity shows some similarities.
- There are limited resources so involvement of the women's groups is essential.
- There may be some non-engagement problems.
- The organisation running the project is similar (health-promotion focused); barriers might include money or language.
- There is a professional physical activity coordinator available, although with a slightly different previous focus.

Transferability criteria indicate:

- There will be a need to investigate prevalence; general statistics indicate approximately one in three women are at risk.
- Some similarities, the women are close in age; there may be some psychological factors that are different, for example, perceived susceptibility and severity.

- Capacity is less in the target setting, and some activities may have to be tailored or adapted – perhaps a shortened programme or different delivery structures.

2 To ensure more success you could involve women's groups in the planning and provision of the programme; consider a pilot study first, and materials may need to be translated.

7.8   Evidence and maternal and child health

1 You might focus on pregnant women, or women post-pregnancy with very small children. Guidance recommends a range of areas such as a focus on breastfeeding, vitamin supplements, liaison with key projects such as Sure Start and appropriate eating (not dieting) during pregnancy. From these data you could select a group like low income pregnant women and then consider how you could implement guidance, e.g. provision of free vitamin supplements, promotion of iron in diet on a low income.

CHAPTER 8

8.1   Who is interested in evaluation and why?

1 The funding organisation, e.g. the local authority, local GPs who have referred, patients, local housing association, community leaders, mental health teams, voluntary groups, programme participants.
2 Fiscal, particularly cost-effectiveness. Quality, assessment of need. Evidence, understanding limitations of the campaign. Policy, to inform future planning.

8.2   Formative evaluation

1 Interviews, with children, teachers, questionnaires, using a needs assessment matrix, school art projects, competitions, photographing favourite foods, keeping food diaries, testing print-based and online media, parent and sibling focus groups.
2 Compare outcomes with current evidence through a systematic literature search and analysis. Investigate environmental determinants and behavioural factors.

8.3   Impact evaluation

1 That drug users accessed the service. The numbers using the service increased. A reduction in needle sharing was reported. More drug users sought help through counselling.

2   Was this impact sustained over a period of time? Did the drug users express their satisfaction with the service? Was it provided at the right time in the right venue? Were the staff able to offer health advice and did this make a difference? For example, has there been a reduction in hepatitis C and HIV rates? Did the programme lead to better health outcomes?

8.4   Well Man clinics

1   Outcome evaluation would cover a wide range of findings in this example. The sample group could be compared with the whole male population or within the low socioeconomic group, for instance:

- Morbidity and mortality of the sample group could be measured in disease such as diabetes, coronary heart disease or cancer.
- The number of men seeking health screening six months later.
- Mean blood pressure and weight could be compared with other groups.
- The numbers stopping smoking over a period of one year or more.
- The take-up of exercise in the target group over a designated period.
- The increase in media articles on men's health issues in Scotland.
- The reduction in STIs.

8.5   Participatory involvement

1   You would probably want evidence of transparency in the decision-making. You would want to trust that the public health advice is accurate and you would want access to relevant information. You may require skills and knowledge to help you cope with the future. You want good access to services. You may not want direct involvement but you will need reassurance that you are represented. The impacts and outcomes of any interventions will need to be shared widely and over a long period of time.
2   Interactive website where concerns can be posted. Attending focus groups, receiving regular public health bulletins. Education and training resources for capacity building to enable people to identify and develop their own needs.

8.6   Ways to evaluate health communication

Accuracy: Were there factual information and key messages about the benefits of participation in sport?

Availability: Was the information available in libraries, GP surgeries, leisure centres, workplaces, websites, local media?

Balance: Were messages about the benefits of sport participation supported by health advice about checking with GP and the availability of appropriate protective equipment or clothing?

Consistency: Did the messages stay the same, were they unambiguous?

Cultural competence: Was consideration given to target groups, for example were they people who already exercised or not? Was gender and ethnicity taken into account?

Evidence base: Were there claims for psychological and physical gains based on reliable studies? Had there been an assessment of need?

Reach: Were there hard-to-reach groups accessed? Were there incentives such as free equipment, competitions, etc.?

Reliability: Was there evidence of a robust planning process and consideration of effectiveness strategies?

Repetition: Were the key messages user-friendly, easily remembered and reinforced across the media?

Timeliness: Was the intervention delivered in a timely fashion?

Understanding: Did the group understand the key messages? Did they understand the information given to them?

8.7   Bullying among young teenagers

1   The findings would be shared with teachers, parents, board of governors and the pupils.

- The teachers may receive written reports, a presentation and possibly a training package or manual.
- Parents of all school children may receive letters, emails or a presentation.
- Parents of the study group may have personal communication or small workshops as well as written information.
- The board of governors would receive a formal evidence-based report and a presentation of findings.
- The pupils may receive information online or through social media; they may have workshops and have a programme integrated into the curriculum.

2   Barriers to dissemination would include:

- The teachers or board of governors may not accept the findings and not want to act on them.
- Parents may not understand the information, there may be language difficulties; the information may not be pitched at the appropriate level for all parents.

- The parents of the children who have been bullied or are bullies may be concerned about confidentiality and not want to participate in any activity.
- The pupils may not be clear what the findings show, they may not understand what bullying constitutes and how it affects people.
- The pupils may not view the findings as important.

GLOSSARY

Agenda setting   Refers to the way the media select events that the public sees and with this selection set the terms of reference for current interest and debate.

Apps   An abbreviation for 'applications' of Games and services that are often connected to the internet available on mobile phones and tablets.

At-risk groups   A group that is vulnerable or susceptible to 'risk' of different types of ill health or disease.

Attitudes   An evaluation that a person makes about an attitude 'object'. The attitude 'object' could be themselves, other people, issues (i.e. in the media) or objects (i.e. alcohol).

Beliefs   The information that a person has about an object or action forms their beliefs.

Bottom-up approach   This proposes that communities or groups know what they want and are involved in all stages of planning and implementing interventions (see Top-down approach).

Brief interventions   A short health promotion session (i.e. 15 minutes) that is designed to prompt behaviour change or challenge attitudes to health-related behaviour.

Bus wraps   A large bill-board style message placed on the outside of a bus.

Campaign   A planned, designed and coordinated effort to promote a particular cause.

Chat rooms   An Internet-based portal where anyone can 'chat' to each other via a mechanism similar to email.

Coalition   An alliance for combined action between populations, parties or groups generally united for a single cause.

Demographics   The characteristics of the population (i.e. social class, age or education) that can be measured via population groups.

Discrimination   The placement of a person below that of another person who does not share the same characteristics (i.e. ethnic group or sex).

E-health   A generic term for all IT applications linked to health and incorporating applications linked to computers, health and medicine that are used to deliver or promote health.

Empowerment A term usually used to describe a way of working that enables people to develop knowledge or skills to increase control and power over life circumstances.

Equity In health, equity is concerned with the differences in health status that are unfair or unequal and the readdressing of these.

Evaluation The process by which worth or value of something is decided involving measurement, observation and comparison with the programme/policy aim.

Evidence-based practice The use of research evidence to guide practice.

Gaming The use of technology (i.e. mobile phones or internet) for game playing purposes. In health promotion these can be games with educational messages or interactions that challenge current practices or enforce current behaviours.

Health advocacy A combination of individual and social actions designed to gain political commitment, support or acceptance.

Health belief model (HBM) A model of behavioural change that focuses on an individual weighing up the risks and benefits of behaviour.

Health Development Agency (HDA) A UK-based specialist health authority that aimed to improve the health of people in England. It has now closed, and has been partly replaced by NICE (see NICE).

Health education Providing information through constructed opportunities that improve knowledge or skills and increase healthy behaviours.

Health promotion The process of enabling people to increase control over their health.

Holism Embodying holistic notions of health (see Holistic).

Holistic A term that includes the wider definition of health including physical, mental, social and spiritual health.

Inequalities (in health) Differences in health status between populations or sections of the population.

IT Information technology, generally includes all interactive media (i.e. CD-ROMs, the Internet, touch-screen kiosks or computers).

Mass media Any type of printed or electronic communication medium that is sent to the population at large.

Model A simplified version of a theoretical construct.

Morbidity The amount of disease there is in a population (i.e. the number of people living with a disease).

Mortality The number of people who have died in the population (i.e. the number of people who have died from certain diseases).

National Service Framework(s) The UK government's long-term strategies for improving different areas of care (i.e. mental health).

NICE The National Institute for Health and Clinical Excellence, the UK's independent health-related organization responsible for providing national guidance on the promotion, prevention and treatment in health.

Ottawa Charter for Health Promotion A World Health Organization policy statement that sets out a clear commitment to health promotion.

Peer education An education method where a person or group with credibility (i.e. older children) work with others (i.e. younger children) to promote health or prevent ill health.

Perceived behavioural control Theoretical model that postulates behaviour can change through a series of steps.

Prevention The avoidance of hazards or risks through the creation of conditions to help avoidance or promote early detection of the hazard or risk.

Prosodic The vocal intonation or rhythmatic aspects of language including pitch or stress placed on words.

Process of behaviour change A step-based model based on the stages a person goes through when making a change in their behaviour.

Public health A societal effort to prevent disease and prolonging life.

Role play An education method where a person 'acts' a response to a situation (i.e. saying 'no' to cigarettes). The audience will then 'model' this same response in a real-life situation.

Screening The procedure for the identification of a certain disease (i.e. breast cancer) to enable early detection and treatment of the disease.

Self-efficacy An individual's judgement of their ability to achieve a certain goal (i.e. stopping smoking).

Settings-based approach Any of a number of locations where people work, play and learn where health can be promoted.

Social media a group of Internet-based applications that allows individuals to create, collaborate, and share content with one another.

SMS messaging 'Short messaging service', the facility and sending of short messages via a mobile phone, more commonly called 'text messaging'.

Stereotyping The act of predicting how another person will act or behave in a certain situation based on preconceived notions of how people act (see Discrimination).

Tablet In IT terms this is a wireless, mobile personal computer with a touchscreen.

Tailoring information   Adapted information for a specific group of people to fit their needs and preferences.

Theory   A set of ideas or arguments that help to understand behaviour in a more simplified way.

Theory of planned behaviour (TPB)   A theoretical model based on the stages a person goes through when changing a behaviour, including perceived behavioural control.

Theory of reasoned action (TRA)   A theoretical model based on the stages a person goes through when changing behaviour; this model is a recent revision of the theory of planned behaviour model.

Top-down approach   An approach which is dictated by those with power that does not directly include the target group or receivers of the intervention (see Bottom-up approach).

Transtheoretical model or 'stages of change' model   A stage-step model based on the stages people go through when making a change in their behaviour.

UNICEF   The United Nations Children's Fund, which has 37 committees world-wide working with, and for, the world's children.

Values   Acquired by the social world, they can influence attitudes and behaviour.

Vignettes   A short impressionistic scene usually with a focus on one version or behaviour at that moment in time.

REFERENCES

Abraham C, Krahe B, Dominic R and Fritsche I (2002) Do health promotion messages target cognitive and behavioural correlates of condom use? A content analysis of safer sex promotion leaflets in two countries. *British Journal of Health Psychology* 7 (2): 227–246.

Abroms LC and Lefebvre RC (2009) Obama's wired campaign: Lessons for public health communication. *Journal of Health Communication* 14 (5): 415–423.

Achterberg T, Huisman-De Waal GGJ, Ketelaar NAB, Oostendorp RA, Jacobs JE and Wollersheim HCH (2010) How to promote healthy behaviors in patients? An overview of evidence for behavior change techniques. *Health Promotion International* 26 (2): 148–162.

Agha S and Beaudoin CE (2012) Assessing thematic condom advertising campaign on condom use in urban Pakistan. *Journal of Health Communication* 24 January [Epub ahead of publication].

Airhihenbuwa CO and Obregon R (2000) A critical assessment of theories/models used in health communication for HIV/AIDS. *Journal of Health Communication* 5 (Suppl.): 5–15.

Ajzen I (1991) The theory of planned behaviour. *Organisational Behaviour and Human Decision Processes* 50: 179–211; available at www.unix.oit.umass.edu/~aizen/index.html, last accessed 16 November 2012.

Ajzen I and Fishbein M (1980) *Understanding Attitudes and Predicting Social Behaviour.* Prentice-Hall, Englewood Cliffs, NJ.

Akhund S and Yousafzai AK (2011) How successful are women's groups in health promotion and disease prevention? A synthesis of the literature and recommendations for developing counties. *Eastern Mediterranean Health Journal* 17 (5): 446–452.

Albrecht K, Simon D, Buchholz A, Reuter K, Frosch D, Seebauer L and Harter M (2011) How does a German audience appraise an American decision aid on early stage breast cancer? *Patient Education and Counseling* 83 (1): 58–63.

Alexander GL, McClure JB, Calvi JH, Divine GW, Stopponi MA, Rolnick SJ, Heimendinger J, Tolsma DD, Resnicow K, Campbell MK, Strecher VJ, Johnson CC and Menu Choices Team (2010) A randomised clinical trial evaluating online interventions to improve fruit and vegetable consumption. *American Journal of Public Health* 100 (2): 319–326.

Alo OA and Gbadebo B (2011) Intergenerational attitude changes regarding female genital cutting in Nigeria. *Journal of Women's Health* 20 (11) 1655–1661.

Andreou G, Gourgoulinis K and Galantomos I (2010) Letter to the editor. The language of the unsuccessful anti-smoking campaign in Greece: Examples from Greek newspaper headlines. *Preventive Medicine* 51 (3–4): 336–337.

Andrews JR, Silk KS and Eneli IU (2010) Parents as health promoters: A theory of planned behavior perspective on the prevention of childhood obesity. *Journal of Health Communication* 15 (1): 95–107.

Angermeyer MC, Holzinger A and Matschinger H (2009) Mental health literacy and attitude towards people with mental illness: A trend analysis based on population surveys in the Eastern part of Germany. *European Psychiatry* 24 (4): 225–232.

Ashbridge M (2006) Public place restrictions on smoking in Canada: Assessing the role of the state, media, science and public health advocacy. *Social Science and Medicine* 58 (1): 13–24.

Askelson NM, Campo S and Carter KD (2011) Completely isolated? Health information seeking among social isolates. *Health Education and Behaviour* 38 (2): 116–122.

Atkin C (2001) Theory and principles of media health campaigns, pp. 49–68 in Rice RE and Atkin CK (eds) *Public Communication Campaigns*, 3rd edition. Sage, London.

Atun RA and Sittampalam SR (2006) A review of the characteristics and benefits of SMS in delivering health care. *The Vodafone Policy Paper Series* 4 (March): 18–28.

Australian Institute of Primary Care (2008) Measuring health promotion impacts: A guide to impact evaluation in integrated health promotion. Rural and Regional Health and Aged Care Service Division, Melbourne.

Ayers JW, Hofstetter CR, Irvin VL, Song Y, Park HR, Paik HY and Hovell MF (2010) Can religion help prevent obesity? Religious messages and the prevalence of being overweight or obese among Korean women in California. *Journal of Scientific Study and Religion* 49 (3): 536–549.

Baker A and Macpherson B (2000) Tomorrow's minds. MIND, London; available at www.mind.org.uk, last accessed 20 April 2012.

Barbor T, Caetano R, Casswell S, Edwards G, Giesbrecht N, Graham K, Giube J, Gruenewald P, Mill L, Holdes M, Homel R, Osterberg E, Rehm J, Roan R and Rossow I (2003) Alcohol – no ordinary commodity. World Health Organization/Society for Addiction, WHO, London.

Baric L (1993) The setting approach – implications for policy and strategy. *Journal of the Institute of Health Education* 31 (1): 17–24.

Baron-Epel O (2010) Attitudes and beliefs associated with mammography in a multiethnic population in Israel. *Health Education and Behaviour* 37 (2): 227–242.

Barretto AI, Bingham CR, Goh KN and Shope JT (2010) Developing a web-based health promotion intervention: A case study from a brief motivational alcohol program. *Health Promotion Practice* 12 (2): 193–201.

Barysch MJ, Cozzio A, Kolm, I, Hrdlicka SR, Brand, C, Hunger R, Kreyden O, Schaffner R, Zaugg T and Crummer R (2010) Internet based health promotion campaign against skin cancer – results of www.skincheck.ch in Switzerland. *European Journal of Dermatology* 20 (1): 109–114.

Bates C, McIntyre D and Watt T (2003) How to run a national tobacco campaign. ASH; available at www.ash.org.uk/files/documents/ASH_205.pdf, last accessed 20 April 2012.

Becker MH (1974) The health belief model and personal health behaviour. *Health Education Monographs* 2 (4): 324–473.

Beiner L, Reimer RL, Wakefield M, Szczypka G, Rigotti NA and Connolly G (2006) Impact of smoking cessation and mass media among recent quitters. *American Journal of Preventive Medicine* 30 (3): 217–224.

Benigeri M and Pluye P (2003) Shortcomings of health information on the internet. *Health Promotion International* 18 (4): 381–386.

Benjamins MR and Brown C (2004) Religion and preventive health care utilization among the elderly. *Social Science and Medicine* 58 (1): 109–111.

Bensberg M and Kennedy M (2002) A framework for health promoting emergency departments. *Health Promotion International* 17 (2): 179–188.

Berger M, Wagner TH and Baker LC (2005) Internet use and stigmatised illness. *Social Science and Medicine* 68 (8): 1821–1827.

Berndt NC, O'Riordan DL, Winkler E, McDermott L, Spathonis K and Owen N (2011) Social cognitive correlates of young adult sport competitors' sunscreen use. *Health Education and Behaviour* 38 (1): 6–14.

Bessinger R, Katende C and Gupta N (2004) Multi-media campaign exposure effects on knowledge and use of condoms for STI and HIV/AIDS prevention in Uganda. *Evaluation and Program Planning* 27 (4): 397–407.

Bish A and Michie S (2010) Demographic and attitudinal determinants of protective behaviours during a pandemic: A review. *British Journal of Health Psychology* 15 (4): 797–824.

Black Barbershop Health Outreach Program (BBHOP) (2012) available at http://blackbarbershop.org/, last accessed 20 April 2012.

Blaxter M (1990) *Health and Lifestyles*. Tavistock/Routledge, London.

Blaxter M (1997) Whose fault is it? People's own conceptions of the reasons for health inequalities. *Social Science and Medicine* 44 (6): 747–756.

Bleakley A, Hennessy M and Jordan A (2011) Using the Integrative Model to explain how exposure to sexual media content influences adolescent sexual behaviour. *Health Education and Behaviour* 38 (5): 530–540.

Bledsoe L (2005) Smoking cessation: An application of theory of planned behaviour to understanding progress through stages of change. *Addictive Behaviours* 30 (7): 1335–1341.

Bopp M and Webb B (2012) Health promotion in megachurches: An untapped resource with megareach? *Health Promotion Practice* 4 April [Epub ahead of publication].

Bradbury H (2009) *Medical Sociology: An introduction*. Sage, London.

Brennan E, Durkin SJ, Cotter T, Harper T and Wakefield MA (2011) Mass media campaigns designed to support new pictorial health warnings on cigarette packets: Evidence of a complementary relationship. *Tobacco Control* 7 April [Epub ahead of publication].

Brice A, Burls A and Hill A (2011) Finding and appraising evidence, pp. 184–193 in Pencheon D, Guest C, Melzer D and Gray JAM (eds) *Oxford Handbook of Public Health Practice*, 2nd edition. Oxford University Press, Oxford.

Brinn MP, Carson KV, Esterman AJ, Chang AB and Smith BJ (2010) Mass media interventions for preventing smoking in young people. *Cochrane Database Systematic Review* 10 (11): CD001006.

British Heart Foundation (BHF) (2012) Hands only CPR; available at www.bhf.org.uk, last accessed 20 April 2012.

Brophy S, Snooks H and Griffiths L (2008) *What is an Evaluation in Small Scale Evaluation in Health: A practical guide*. Sage, London.

Brown A and Lee M (2011) An exploration of the attitudes and experience of mothers in the United Kingdom who chose to breastfeed exclusively for 6 months postpartum. *Breastfeeding Medicine* 6 August: 197–204.

Browne J (2010) Securing a sustainable future for higher education: An independent review of higher education funding and student finance; available at www.bis.gov.uk/assets/biscore/corporate/docs/s/10-1208-securing-sustainable-higher-education-browne-report.pdf, last accessed 20 April 2012.

Brug J, Conner M, Harré N, Kremers S, McKeller S and Whitelaw S (2005) The transtheoretical model of change: A critique. *Health Education Research* 20 (2): 244–258.

Bruga R, Balfe M, Jeffares I, Conroy RN, Clarke E, Fitzgerald M, O'Donnell E, Vaughan D, Coleman, C, McGee H, Gillespie P and O'Donovan D (2011) Where do young adults want opportunistic chlamydia screening services to be located? *Journal of Public Health* 33 (4): 571–578.

Bryson JM, Quinn Patton M and Bowman RA (2011) Working with evaluation stakeholders: A rationale, step-wise approach and toolkit. *Evaluation and Programme Planning* 34: 1–12.

Buchthal OV, Doff AL, Hsu LA, Silbanuz A, Heinrich KM and Maddock JE (2011) Avoiding a knowledge gap in a multi-ethnic statewide social marketing campaign: Is cultural tailoring sufficient? *Journal of Health Communication* 16 (3): 314–327.

Buller DB, Woodhall WG, Hall JR, Borland R, Ax B, Brown M and Hines JM (2001) A web-based smoking cessation and prevention program for children aged 12–15, pp. 357–372 in

Rice RE and Aktin CK (eds) *Public Communication Campaigns*, 3rd edition. Sage, Thousand Oaks, CA.

Burke RC, Wilson J, Kowalski A, Murrill C, Cutler C, Sweeney M and Begier EM (2011) NYC condoms use and satisfaction and demand for alternative condom products in New York City sexually transmitted disease clinics. *Journal of Urban Health* 88 (4): 749–758.

Burns ME, See Tai S, Lai R and Nazareth I (2006) Interactive health communication applications for people with chronic disease (review). *Cochrane Database of Systematic Reviews* 19 (4): CD004274.

Byrd TL, Peterson SK, Chavez R and Heckert A (2004) Cervical screening beliefs among young Hispanic women. *Preventive Medicine* 38 (2): 192–197.

Callaghan P, Khalil E and Morres I (2010) A prospective evaluation of the Transtheoretical Model of Change applied to exercise in young people. *International Journal of Nursing Studies* 47 (1): 3–12.

Campbell MK, Hudson MA, Resnicow K, Blakeney N, Paxton A and Baskin M (2009) Church-based health promotion interventions: Evidence and lessons learned; available at http://nysdiabetes.forumone.com/userfiles/Church-Based-Health-Promotion-Interventions_Evidence-and-Lessons-Learned.pdf, last accessed 20 April 2012.

Campbell MK, James A, Hudson MA, Carr C, Jackson E, Oates V, Demissie S, Farrell D and Tessaro I (2004) Improving multiple behaviours for colorectal cancer prevention among African American church members. *Health Psychology* 23 (5): 492–502.

Cancer Research UK (2009) Policy statement: Sunbeds; available at http://info.cancerresearchuk.org/prod_consump/groups/cr_common/@nre/@sta/documents/generalcontent/014390.pdf, last accessed 20 April 2012.

Caprio S, Daniels SR, Drewnowski A, Kaufman FR, Palinkas LA, Rosenbloom AL, Schwimmer JB (2008) Influence of race, ethnicity and culture on childhood obesity: Implications for prevention and treatment. *Diabetes Care* 31 (11): 2211–2220.

Card JJ, Solomon J and Cunningham SD (2011) How to adapt effective programs for use in new contexts. *Health Promotion Practice* 12 (1): 25–35.

Cashen MS, Dykes P and Gerber B (2004) E-health technology and Internet resources: Barriers for vulnerable population. *Journal of Cardiovascular Nursing* 19 (3): 209–214.

Cassell MM, Jackson C and Cheuvront B (1998) Health communication on the Internet: An effective channel for behaviour change? *Journal of Health Communication* 3 (1): 71–79.

Cates JR, Shafer A, Diehl SJ and Deal AM (2011) Evaluating a county-sponsored social marketing campaign to increase mothers' initiative of HPV vaccine for their pre-teen daughters in a primarily rural area. *Social Marketing Quarterly* 17 (1): 4–26.

Cavill N, Buxton K, Bull F and Foster C (2006) Promotion of physical activity among adults, evidence into practice briefing. NICE, London; available at www.nice.org.uk/niceMedia/pdf/physical_activity_eip_v3.pdf, last accessed 20 April 2012.

Center for Chronic Disease Prevention and Health Promotion (CDC) (2009) Evaluation briefs: Developing process evaluation questions. No. 4; available at www.cdc.gov/healthyyouth/evaluation/pdf/brief4.pdf, last accessed 20 April 2012.

Centre for Chronic Disease Prevention and Health Promotion (CDC) (2012) *Right to Know*; available at www.cdc.gov/ncbddd/disabilityandhealth/righttoknow/, last accessed 16 November 2012.

Center for Communication Programs (CCP) (2003) A field guide to designing a health communication strategy. Johns Hopkins University; available at www.jhuccp.org, last accessed 20 April 2012.

Char A, Saavala M and Kulmala T (2011) Assessing young unmarried men's access to reproductive health information and services in rural India. *BMC Public Health* 17 (11): 476.

Charities Evaluation Service (2012) available at www.ces-vol.org.uk, last accessed 20 April 2012.

Chiao C, Mishra V and Ksobiech K (2011) Spousal communication about HIV prevention in Kenya. *Journal of Health Communication* 16 (10): 1088–1105.

Cho H and Choi J (2010) Predictors and the role of attitude toward the message and perceived message quality in gain- and loss-frame antidrug persuasion of adolescents. *Health Communication* 25 (4): 303–311.

Chivu CM and Reidpath DD (2010) Social deprivation and exposure to health promotion: A study of the distribution of health promotion resources to schools in England. *BMC Public Health* 10: 473.

Christensen CL, Bowen DJ, Hart A, Kuniyuki A, Saleeba AE and Kramish Campbell M (2005) Recruitment of religious organizations into a community-based health promotion programme. *Health and Social Care in the Community* 13 (4): 313–322.

Clayman ML, Manganello JA, Viswanath K, Hesse BW and Arora NK (2010) Providing health messages to Hispanics/Latinos: Understanding the importance of language, trust in health information sources, and media use. *Journal of Health Communication* 15 (Suppl. 3): 252–263.

Cline RJW and Haynes KM (2001) Consumer health information seeking on the Internet: The state of the art. *Health Education Research* 16 (6): 671–692.

Coombes Y (2010) Feeding back evaluation results to stakeholder participants, in Thorogood M and Coombes Y (eds) (2010) *Evaluating Health Promotion: Practice and methods*, 3rd edition. Oxford University Press, Oxford, p. 187–196.

Corcoran N (2011) *Working on Health Communication*. Sage, London.

Cornwall and the Isles of Scilly Health Authority (1999) Bones in Mind osteoporosis project. Cornwall and IOS HP Department, Cornwall.

Cottrell L, Harris CV, Deskins S, Bradlyn A and Coffman JW (2010) Developing culturally tailored health belief-based intervention materials to improve child and parent participation in a cardiovascular screening program. *Health Promotion Practice* 11 (3): 418–427.

Creel AH, Rimal RN, Mkandawire G, Bose K and Brown JW (2011) Effects of a mass media intervention on HIV related stigma: 'Radio Diaries' program in Malawi. *Health Education Research* 26 (3): 456–465.

Cugelman B, Thelwall M and Dawes P (2011) Online interventions for social marketing health behavior change campaigns: A meta analysis of psychological architectures and adherence factors. *Journal of Medical Internet Research* 13 (1): e17.

Cummins S and Macintyre S (2002) 'Food deserts' – evidence and assumptions in health policy making. *British Medical Journal* 325: 436–438.

Da Costa TM, Salomao PL, Martha AS, Pisa IT and Sigulem D (2010) The impact of short message service text messages sent as appointment reminders to patients call phones at outpatients clinics in Sao Paulo, Brazil. *International Journal Medical Information* 79 (1): 65–70.

Dale R and Hanbury A (2010) A simple methodology for piloting and evaluating mass media interventions: An exploratory study. *Psychology, Health and Medicine* 15 (2): 231–242.

Darker CD, French DP, Eves FF and Sniehotta FF (2010) An intervention to promote walking amongst the general population based on an extended theory of planned behaviour: A waiting list randomised controlled trial. *Psychology and Health* 25 (1): 71–88.

De Leeuw E (2011) Do healthy cities work? A logic of method for assessing impact and outcome of healthy cities. *Journal of Urban Health* 89 (2): 1–15.

Department for Education and Skills (DfES) (2004) *Healthy Living Blueprint for Schools*. The Stationery Office, London.

Department for Transport (DfT) (2012a) Interactive driving challenge; available at http:// think.direct.gov.uk/, last accessed 20 April 2012.

Department for Transport (DfT) (2012b) Tales of the Road; available at www.talesoftheroad. direct.gov.uk, last accessed 20 April 2012.

Department for Transport (DfT) (2012c) *Think Bike. Think Biker*; available at www.think. direct.gov.uk/motorcycles.html, last accessed 16 November 2012.

Department of Health (DH) (1992) *The Health of the Nation*. HMSO, London.

Department of Health (DH) (2001) *National Service Framework for Older People*. The Stationery Office, London.

Department of Health (DH) (2004) *Choosing Health: Making healthy choices easier*. The Stationery Office, London.

Department of Health (DH) (2008) COI Research Management Summary on Behalf of the Department of Health Chlamydia Screening and Sexual Health Marketing – Research with Young People conducted by Define available at www.dh.gov.uk/prod_consum_dh/groups/dh_ digitalassets/@dh/@en/documents/digitalasset/dh_114607.pdf, last accessed 20 August 2012.

Department of Health (DH) (2009a) Change4Life; available at www.nhs.uk/Change4Life/, last accessed 20 April 2012.

Department of Health (DH) (2009b) Sex Worth Talking About campaign toolkit; available at www.nhs.uk/sexualhealthprofessional/Documents/SWTA_campaign_toolkit_final.pdf, last accessed 20 April 2012.

Department of Health (DH) (2010a) Healthy lives, healthy people: Our strategy for public health in England; available at www.dh.gov.uk, last accessed 20 April 2012.

Department of Health (DH) (2010b) Change4Life convenience stores evaluation report: Promoting the purchase of fresh fruit and vegetables in deprived areas; available at www. dh.gov.uk/prod_consum_dh/groups/dh_digitalassets/@dh/@en/@ps/documents/digitalasset/ dh_120801.pdf, last accessed 20 April 2012.

Department of Health (DH) (2012) Bowel Cancer Campaign Second Phase Launched; available at http://campaigns.dh.gov.uk/2012/08/27/be-clear-on-cancer-leaflet

De Wit JBF, Vef R, Schutten M and Van Steenbergen J (2005) Social-cognitive determinants of vaccination behaviour against hepatitis B: An assessment among men who have sex with men. *Preventive Medicine* 40 (6): 795–802.

Diedrichs PC, Lee C and Kelly M (2011) Seeing the beauty in everyday people: A qualitative study of young Australians' opinions on body image, the mass media and models. *Body Image* 8 (3): 259–266.

Di Noia J and Prochaska JO (2010) Mediating variables in a transtheoretical model dietary intervention program. *Health Education and Behaviour* 37 (5): 753–762.

Di Noia J, Contento IR and Prochaska JO (2008) Computer mediated intervention tailored on transtheoretical model stages and processes of change increases fruit and vegetable consumption among urban African-American adolescents. *American Journal of Health Promotion* 22 (5): 336–341.

Dooris M (2001) Health promoting universities: Policy and practice: a UK perspective. CCPH 2001 conference papers; available at www.depts.washington.edu/ccph/pdf_files/p-dooris.pdf.

Dooris M (2005) Healthy settings: Challenges to generating evidence of effectiveness. *Health Promotion International* 21 (1): 55–65.

Dooris M and Doherty S (2009) National Research and Development Project on Healthy Universities; available at www.hsaparchive.org.uk/rp/publications/projectreports/2009mdooris. pdf, last accessed 20 April 2012.

Dooris M and Thompson J (2001) Health-promoting universities: An overview, pp. 156–168 in Scriven A and Orme J (2001) *Health Promotion Professional Perspectives*. Palgrave, Basingstoke.

Downie RS, Fyfe C and Tannahill A (1992) *Health Promotion: Models and Values.* Oxford University Press, Oxford.

Downing-Matibag TM and Geisinger R (2009) Hooking up and sexual risk taking among college students: A health belief model perspective. *Qualitative Health Research* 19 (9): 1196–1209.

Drummond MF, Sculpher MJ, Torrance GW, O'Brien BJ and Stoddart GL (2005) *Methods for Economic Evaluation of Health Care Programmes*, 3rd edition. Oxford University Press, Oxford.

Duan N, Fox S, Pitkin K, Derose K, Carson S and Stockdale S (2005) Identifying churches for community-based mammography promotion: Lessons from the LAMP study. *Health Education and Behaviour* 32 (4): 536–548.

Duffy M, Wimbush E, Reece J and Eadie D (2002) Net profits? Web site development and health improvement. *Health Education* 103 (5): 278–285.

Dunne C and Somerset M (2004) Health promotion in university: What do students want? *Health Education* 104 (6): 360–367.

Dunn KL, Mohr P, Wilson CJ and Wittert GA (2011) Determinants of fast-food consumption: An application of the theory of planned behavior. *Appetite* 57 (2): 349–357.

ECDC (2011) Evidence-based methodologies for public health. ECDC, Stockholm; available at www.ecdc.europa.eu/en/publications/Publications/1109_TER_evidence_based_methods_for_public_health.pdf, last accessed 20 April 2012.

Elder JP (2001) *Behaviour Change and Public Health in the Developing World.* Sage, London.

Elliott MA and Armitage CJ (2009) Promoting drivers' compliance with speed limits: Testing an intervention based on the theory of planned behaviour. *British Journal of Psychology* 100 (1): 111–132.

Ellis A and Beattie G (1986) *The Psychology of Language and Communication.* Laurence Erlbaum, London.

Evenson KR and Bradley CB (2010) Beliefs about exercise and physical activity among pregnant women. *Patient Education and Counseling* 79 (1): 124–129.

Eysenbach G (2001) What is e-health? *Journal of Medical Internet Research* 3 (2); available at www.jmir.org/2001/2/e20/, last accessed 20 April 2012.

Farrelly MC, Niederdeppe J and Yarsevich J (2003) Youth tobacco prevention mass media campaigns: Past, present, and future directions. *Tobacco Control* 12 (Suppl. 1): i35–i47.

Fernando S (2003) *Cultural Diversity, Mental Health and Psychiatry.* Routledge, London.

Ferrante JM, Shaw EK and Scott JG (2011) Factors influencing men's decisions regarding prostate cancer screening: A qualitative study. *Journal of Community Health* 36 (5): 839–844.

Fertman CI and Allensworth DD (eds) (2010) *Health Promotion Programmes: From theory to practice.* Jossey Bass, San Francisco.

Fishbein M and Capella JN (2006) The role of theory in developing effective health communications. *Journal of Communication* 56 (S1): S1–S17.

Fors M and Moreno A (2002) The benefits and obstacles of implementing ICTs strategies for development from a bottom-up approach. *Aslib Proceedings* 54 (3): 198–206; available at www.emeraldinsight.com, last accessed 16 November 2012.

Freudenberg N (2005) Public health advocacy to change corporate practices: Implications for health education practice and research. *Health Education and Behaviour* 32 (3): 298–319.

Freudenburg N, Bradley SP and Serrano M (2009) Public health campaigns to change industry practices that damage health: An analysis of 12 case studies. *Health Education and Behaviour* 36 (2): 230–249.

Gagnon M, Jacob JD and Holmes D (2010) Governing through (in)security: A critical analysis of a fear-based public health campaign. *Critical Public Health* 20 (2): 245–256.

Gainer E, Sollet C, Ulmann M, Levy D and Ulmann A (2003) Surfing on the morning after: Analysis of an emergency contraception website. *Contraception* 67 (3): 195–199.

Galarce EM, Ramanadhan S, Weeks S, Schneider EC, Gray SW and Viswanath K (2011) Class, race, ethnicity and information needs in post-treatment cancer patients. *Patient Education and Counseling* 85 (3): 432–439.

Gibson DR, Zhang G, Pappas L, Mitchell J and Kegeles SM (2010) Effectiveness of HIV prevention social marketing with injecting drug users. *American Journal of Public Health* 100 (10): 1828–1831.

Glanz K and Yaroch AL (2004) Strategies for increasing fruit and vegetable intake in grocery stores and communities: Policy, pricing and environmental change. *Preventive Medicine* 39 (Suppl. 1): S75–S80.

Global Monitoring Media Project (GMMP) (2010) Who makes the news? available at www.awcfs.org/dmdocuments/reports/gmmp_global_report_en.pdf.

Gorsky M, Krajewski-siuda K, Duta W and Berridge V (2010) Anti-alcohol posters in Poland 1945–1989: Diverse meanings, uncertain effects. *American Journal of Public Health* 100 (11): 2059–2069.

Gould D (2004) Writing a media analysis; available at www.mediaevaluationproject.org/workingpaper2, last accessed 20 April 2012.

Graff M, Davies J and McNorton M (2004) Cognitive style and cross-cultural differences in Internet use and computer attitudes. *European Journal of Open, Distance and E-Learning* (II); available at www.eurodl.org.

Green EC and Witte K (2006) Can fear arousal in public health campaigns contribute to the decline of HIV prevalence? *Journal of Health Communication* 11 (3): 245–259.

Green J and Tones K (2011) *Health Promotion Planning and Strategies*, 2nd edition. Sage, London.

Grier S and Bryant CA (2005) Social marketing in public health. *Annual Review Public Health* 26 (1): 319–339.

Griffith C, Johnson AM, Fenton KA, Erens B, Hart GJ, Wellings K and Mercer CH (2011) Attitudes and first heterosexual experiences among Indians and Pakistanis in Britain: Evidence from a national probability survey. *International Journal of Sexually Transmitted Disease and AIDS* 22 (3): 131–139.

Grilli R, Ramsey C and Minozzi S (2006) Mass media interventions: Effects in health services utilization. *Cochrane Database of Systematic Reviews* 1: CD000389.

Guida GF (2010) Mass media and communication. Council for Cardiology Practice news editorial; available at www.escardio.org, last accessed 20 April 2012.

Hale JL and Dillard JP (1995) Fear appeals in health promotion campaigns: Too much, too little, or just right? pp. 65–80 in Maibach E and Parrott RL (eds) *Designing Health Messages*. Sage, London.

Hall IJ, Johnson-Turbes A and Williams KN (2010) The potential of black radio to dissemination health messages and reduce disparities. Centers for Disease Control and Prevention (CDC); available at www.cdc.gov/pcd/issues/2010/jul/09_0194/htm, last accessed 16 November 2012.

Hall J and Visser A (2000) Health communication in the century of the patient (Editorial). *Patient Education and Counseling* 41 (1): 115–116.

Hamel LM, Robbins LB and Wilbur J (2010) Computer and web-based interventions to increase preadolescent and adolescent physical activity: A systematic review. *Journal of Advanced Nursing* 67 (2): 251–268.

Hanks AS, Just DR, Smith LE and Wansink B (2012) Healthy convenience: Nudging students toward healthier choices in the lunchroom. *Journal of Public Health* 31 January [Epub ahead of publication].

Harrabin R, Coote A and Allen J (2003) *Health in the News*. Kings Fund Publications, London; available at www.kingsfund.org.uk/publications.

Harris JR, Cheadle A, Hannon PA, Forehand M, Lichiello P, Mahoney E, Snyder S and Yarrow JA (2012) Framework for disseminating evidence-based health promotion practices. Prevention of Chronic Diseases 9; available at www.cdc.gov/pcd/issues/2012/11_0081.htm, last accessed 20 April 2012.

Harrison T (2003) Evidence-based multidisciplinary public health, pp. 228–245 in Orme J, Powell J, Taylor P, Harrison T and Grey M (eds) *Public Health for the 21st Century*. Open University Press, Buckingham.

Haug S, Meyer C, Ulbricht S, Schorr G, Rüge J, Rumpf HJ and John U (2010) Predictors and moderators of outcome in different brief interventions for smoking cessation in general medical practice. *Patient Education and Counselling* 78 (1): 57–64.

Health Development Agency (HDA) (2004) The effectiveness of public health campaigns. HDA Briefing 7; available at www.nice.org.uk/niceMedia/documents/CHB7-campaigns-14-7.pdf, last accessed 20 April 2012.

Health Development Agency (HDA) (2005) *HDA Evidence Base, Process and Quality Standards Manual for Evidence Briefings*, 3rd edition. Health Development Agency, London.

Healthy Universities (2011) Communicating health as part of a whole system healthy universities approach; available at www.healthyuniversities.ac.uk/toolkit/uploads/files/communicating_health_messages_guidance_package.pdf, last accessed 20 April 2012.

Henley N and Donovan RJ (2003) Young people's responses to death threat appeals: Do they really feel immortal? *Health Education Research* 18 (1): 1–14.

Hesse BW, Johnson LE and Davis KL (2010) Editorial: Extending the reach, effectiveness, and efficiency of communication: Evidence from the centers of excellence in cancer communication research. *Patient Education and Counseling* 81 (Suppl.): S1–S5.

Hill EK, Alpi KM and Auerbach M (2010) Evidence-based practice in health education and promotion: A review and introduction to resources. *Health Promotion Practice* 11 (3): 358–366.

Hill L (2004) Alcohol promotion via mass media: The evidence on (in)effectiveness. Eurocare 'Bridging the Gap' conference report, Warsaw; available at www.eurocare.org.

Hills M and McQueen DV (2007) At issue: Two decades of the Ottawa Charter. *International Journal of Health Promotion and Education* Special edition 2; available at www.iuhpe.org/upload/File/PE_Ottawa_07a.pdf, last accessed 20 April 2012.

Hoek J, Wilson N, Allen M, Edwards R, Thomson G and Li J (2010) Lessons from New Zealand's introduction of pictorial health warnings on tobacco packaging. *Bulletin of the World Health Organization* 88: 861–866.

Hogan DR, Baltussen R, Hayashi C, Lauer JA and Salomon JA (2005) Cost effectiveness analysis of strategies to combat HIV/AIDs in developing countries. *British Medical Journal* 331 (17): 1431–1435.

Holmberg C, Harttig U, Schulze MB and Boeing H (2011) The potential of the Internet for health communication: The use of an interactive on-line tool for diabetes risk predictions. *Patient Education and Counseling* 83 (1): 106–112.

Holmes D (2010) Campaigns: Celebrities and cancer campaigns: Time for a re-think? *The Lancet* 11 (4): 320.

Hopman-Rock M, Bourghouts JAJ and Leurs MTW (2004) Determinants of participation in a health education and exercise program on television. *Preventive Medicine* 41 (3): 232–239.

Horvath KJ, Harwood EM, Courtenay-Quirk C, McFarlane M, Fisher H, Dickenson T, Kachur R and Rosser BRS (2010) Online resources for persons recently diagnosed with HIV/AIDs: An analysis of HIV-related webpages. *Journal of Health Communication* 15 (5): 516–531.

House of Commons (2012) *Population ageing*. Statistics available at www.parliament.uk/briefing-papers/SN03228.pdf last accessed 20 August 2012.

House of Commons Health Committee (2009) *Health Inequalities 2008–9 Third Report*, Vol. 1. The Stationery Office, London.

Hughner R and Kleine S (2004) Views of health in the lay sector: A compilation and review of how individuals think about health. *Health* 8 (4): 395–422.

Huhman ME, Potter LD, Nolin MJ, Piesse A, Judkins DR, Banspach SW and Wong FL (2010) The influence of the VERB campaign on children's physical activity in 2002 to 2006. *American Journal of Public Health* 100 (4): 635–683.

Humphrys J (2012) Billboard behaviours as part of BBC Radio 4's Today Programme; available at www.bbc.co.uk/news/world-africa-17668616, last accessed 20 April 2012.

Hutchison AJ, Breckon JD and Johnston LH (2009) Physical activity behaviour change interventions based on the transtheoretical model: A systematic review. *Health Education and Behaviour* 36 (5): 829–845.

Huttner B, Goossens H, Verheji T and Harbarth S (2010) Characteristics and outcomes of public campaigns aimed at improving the use of antibiotics in outpatients in high income countries. *The Lancet Infectious Diseases* 10 (1): 17–31.

Improvement and Development Agency (2011) Get a new hair cut and a new mental attitude; available at www.idea.gov.uk/idk/core/page.do?pageId=25067289, last accessed 20 April 2012.

Jack L (2010) Health promotion practice and the next 5 years: Thoughts from the newly appointed editor-in-chief. *Health Promotion Practice* 11 (1): 5–6.

Jackson C, Lawton R, Knapp P, Raynor DK, Connor M, Lowe C and Closs SJ (2005) Beyond intention: Do specific plans increase health behaviours in patients in primary care? A study of fruit and vegetable consumption. *Social Science and Medicine* 60 (10): 2383–2391.

Jacobs EA, Karavolos K, Rathouz PJ, Ferris TG and Powell LH (2005) Limited English proficiency and breast and cervical screening in a multi-ethnic population. *American Journal of Public Health* 95 (8): 1410–1416.

Jamieson A (2002) Theory and practice in social gerontology, pp. 7–20 in Jamieson A and Victor C (eds) *Researching Ageing and Later Life*. Open University Press, Buckingham.

Janz NK and Becker MH (1984) The health belief model a decade later. *Health Education Quarterly* 11 (1): 1–47.

Johnson J (2011) 10 apps for counting calories; available at http://iphone.appstorm.net/roundups/lifestyle-roundups/10-iphone-apps-for-counting-calories/, last accessed 20 April 2012.

Jones RK and Biddlecom AE (2011) Is the internet filling the sexual health information gap for teens? An exploratory study. *Journal of Health Communication* 16 (2): 112–123.

Jones S and Donovan RJ (2004) Does theory inform practice in health promotion in Australia? *Health Education Research* 19 (1): 1–14.

Kakai H, Maskarinec G, Shumay DM, Tatsumura Y and Tasaki K (2003) Ethnic difference in choices of health information by cancer patients using complementary and alternative medicine: An exploratory study with correspondence analysis. *Social Science and Medicine* 56 (2): 851–862.

Kamiya K (2012) Health management and future activities of Fukushima Prefecture. Seminar on Fukushima Reconstruction, Japan; available at www.iae.or.jp/jyosen/pdf/Fukushima (Feb_4th)/16_KAMIYA(Japan)/Prof_Kamiya(Japan)_English.pdf, last accessed 20 April 2012.

Katz J and Lazarsfeld E (1955) *Personal Influence*. Free Press, New York.

Katz J, Perbedy A and Douglas J (eds) (2000) *Promoting Health: Knowledge and practice*. Palgrave Macmillan, Basingstoke.

Kemp GA, Eagle L and Verne J (2011) Mass media barriers to social marketing interventions: The example of sun protection in the UK. *Health Promotion International* 26 (1): 37–45.

Kharbanda EO, Stockwell MS, Fox HW, Andres R, Lara M and Rickert VI (2011) Text message reminders to promote human papillomavirus vaccination. *Vaccine* 29 (14): 2537–2541.

Khowaja LA, Khuwaja AK, Nayani P, Jessani S, Khowaja MP and Khowaja S (2010) Quit smoking for life – social marketing strategy for young: A case for Pakistan. *Journal of Cancer Education* 25 (4): 637–642.

King R, Estey J, Allen S, Kegeles S, Wolf W, Valentine C and Sefufilira A (1995) A family planning intervention to reduce vertical transmission of HIV in Rwanda. *AIDS* 9 (Suppl. 1): 45–51.

Kirigia JM, Seddoh A, Gatwiri D, Muthuri LHK and Seddoh J (2005) E-health: Determinants, opportunities, challenges and the way forward for countries in the WHO Africa region. *BMC Public Health* 5 (137); available at www.biomedcentral.com/1471–2458/5/137, last accessed 20 April 2012

Kirk A, MacMillan F and Webster N (2010) Application of the Transtheoretical Model to physical activity in older adults with Type 2 diabetes and/or cardiovascular disease. *Psychology of Sport and Exercise* 11 (4): 320–324.

Knai C, Pomerleau J, Lock K and McKee M (2006) Getting children to eat more fruit and vegetables: A systematic review. *Preventive Medicine* 42 (2): 85–95.

Knerr W (2011) Does condom social marketing improve health outcomes and increase usage and equitable access? *Reproductive Health Matters* 19 (37): 166–173.

Kobetz E, Vatalaro K, Moore A and Earp JA (2005) Taking the transtheoretical model into the field: A curriculum for lay health advisors. *Health Promotion Practice* 6 (3): 329–337.

Koch-Weser S, Bradshaw YS, Gualtieri L and Gallagher SS (2010) The internet as a health information source: Findings from the 2007 health information national trends survey and implications for health communication. *Journal of Health Communication* 15 (Suppl. 3): 279–293.

Koehly LM, Peters JA, Kenen R, Hoskins LM, Ersig AL, Khun NR, Loud JT and Greene MH (2009) Characteristics of health information gatherers, disseminators and blockers with families at risk of hereditary cancer: Implications for family health communication interventions. *American Journal of Public Health* 99 (12): 2203–2209.

Korp P (2006) Health on the Internet: Implications for health promotion. *Health Education Research* 21 (1): 78–86.

Kothe EJ, Millan BA and Amaratunga R (2011) Randomised controlled trial of a brief theory-based intervention promoting breakfast consumption. *Appetite* 56 (1): 148–155.

Kotler JA, Schiffman JM and Hanson KG (2012) The influence of media characters on children's food choices. *Journal of Health Communication* 4 April [Epub ahead of publication].

Kreps GL (2003) The impact of communication on cancer risk, incidence, morbidity, mortality and quality of life. *Health Communication* 15 (2): 161–169.

Kreps GL (2012) Translating health communication research into practice: The importance of implementing and sustaining evidence-based health communication interventions. *Atlantic Communication Journal* 20 (1): 5–15.

Kreps GL and Maibach EW (2008) Transdisciplinary science: The nexus between communication and public health. *Journal of Communication* 58 (4): 732–748.

Kreps GL and Neuhauser L (2010) New directions in eHealth communication: Opportunities and challenges. *Patient Education and Counseling* 78 (2010): 329–336.

Kreps GL and Sparks L (2008) Meeting the health literacy needs of immigrant populations. *Patient Education and Counseling* 71 (3): 328–332.

Kreuter MW, Lukwago SN, Bucholtz DC, Clarke EM and Sanders-Thompson V (2003) Achieving cultural appropriateness in health promotion programs: Targeted and tailored approaches. *Health Education and Behaviour* 30 (2): 133–146.

Kulukulualani M, Braun KL, Tsark JU (2008) Using a participatory four step protocol to develop culturally targeted cancer education brochures. *Health Promotion Practice* 9 (4): 344–55.

Lajunen T and Räsänen M (2004) Can social psychological models be used to promote bicycle helmet use among teenagers? A comparison of the health belief model, theory of planned behaviour and the locus of control. *Journal of Safety Research* 35 (1): 115–123.

Lancaster R and Ward R (2002) Management of work-related road safety. Report for HSE/Scottish Executive. The Stationery Office, Norwich; available at www.hse.gov.uk

Langille JD, Berry TR, Reade IL, Witcher C, Loitz CC and Rodgers WM (2011) Strength of messaging in changing attitudes in a workplace wellness program. *Health Promotion Practice* 12 (2): 303–311.

Latimer AE, Krishnan-Sarin S, Cavallo DA, Duhig A, Salovey P and O'Malley SA (2012) Targeted smoking cessation messages for adolescents. *Journal of Adolescent Health* 50 (1): 47–53.

Lavin D and Groarke A (2005) Dental-floss behaviour: A test of the predictive utility of the theory of planned behaviour and the effects of making implementation interventions. *Psychology, Health and Medicine* 10 (3): 243–252.

Leake AR, Bermudo VC, Jacob J, Jacob MR and Inouye J (2011) Health is wealth: Methods to improve attendance in a lifestyle intervention for a largely immigrant Filipino-American sample. *Journal of Immigrant and Minority Health* 7 June [Epub ahead of publication].

Lee JT, Tsai JL, Tsou TS andChen MC (2011) Effectiveness of a theory-based postpartum sexual health education program on women's contraceptive use: a randomized controlled trial. *Contraception* 84 (1): 48–56.

Lee RG and Garvin T (2003) Moving from information transfer to information exchange in health and health care. *Social Science and Medicine* 56 (3): 449–464.

Levandowski BA, Sharma P, Lane SD, Webster N, Nestor AM, Cibula DA and Huntington S (2006) Parental literacy and infant health: An evidence-based health start intervention. *Health Promotion Practice* 7 (1): 95–102.

Levin J and Hein JF (2012) A faith-based prescription for the surgeon general: Challenges and recommendations. *Journal of Religion and Health* 51 (1): 57–71.

Lewin K (1951) *Field Theory in Social Science: Selected theoretical papers.* Harper Row, New York.

Lewis YR, Shain L, Quinn SC, Turner K and Moore T (2002) Building community trust: Lessons from an STD/HIV peer educator program with African American barbers and beauticians. *Health Promotion Practice* 3 (2): 133–143.

Liang W, Wang J, Chen M, Feng S, Yi B and Mandelblatt JS (2009) Cultural views, language ability, and mammography use in Chinese American women. *Health Education and Behaviour* 36 (6): 1012–1020.

Lieberman DA (2001) Using interactive media in communication campaigns for children and adolescents, pp. 373–388 in Rice RE and Aktin CK (eds) *Public Communication Campaigns*, 3rd edition. Sage, Thousand Oaks, CA.

Lin P, Simoni JM and Zemon V (2005) The health belief model, sexual behaviours and HIV risk among Taiwanese immigrants. *Aids Education and Research* 17 (5): 469–483.

Lin W, Yang H, Hang C and Pan W (2007) Nutrition knowledge, attitude and behaviour of Taiwanese elementary school children. *Asian Pacific Journal of Clinical Nutrition* 16 (Suppl. 2): 534–546.

Lindsay S, King G, Klassen AF, Esses V and Stachel M (2012) Working with immigrant families raising a child with a disability: Challenges and recommendations for healthcare and community service providers. *Disability Rehabilitation* 29 March [Epub ahead of publication].

Linnan LA and Ferguson YO (2007) Beauty salons: A promising health promotion setting for reaching and promoting health among African American women. *Health Education and Behaviour* 34 (3): 517–530.

Linnan LA, Kim AE, Wasilewski Y, Lee AM, Yang J and Solomon F (2001) Working with licensed cosmetologists to promote health: Results from the North Carolina BEAUTY and health pilot study. *Preventive Medicine* 33 (6): 606–612.

Linnan LA, Owens Ferguson Y, Wasilewski Y, Lee AM, Yang J, Solomon F and Katz M (2005) Using community-based participatory research methods to reach women with health messages: Results from the North Carolina BEAUTY and health pilot project. *Health Promotion Practice* 6 (2): 164–173.

Linnan LA, Reiter PL, Duffy C, Hales D, Ward DS and Viera AJ (2011) Assessing and promoting physical activity in African American barbershops: Results of the FITStop pilot study. *American Journal of Men's Health* 5 (1): 38–46.

Lochard J (2004) Living in contaminated territories: A lesson in stakeholder involvement. Centre d'etude sur l'evaluation de la protection dans la domaine Nucleaire (CEPN) France; available at http://irpa11.irpa.net/pdfs/KL-9b.pdf, last accessed 20 April 2012.

Longfield K, Panvanouvong X, Chen J and Kays MB (2011) Increasing safer sexual behavior among Lao kathoy through an intergrated social marketing approach. *BMC Public Health* 11: 872.

Ma M, Dollar KM, Kibler JL, Sarpong D and Samuels D (2011) The effects of priming on a public health campaign targeting cardiovascular risks. *Prevention Science* 12 (3): 333–338.

Macdonald G and Davies JK (2007) Reflection and vision: Proving and improving the promotion of health, in Davis JK and Macdonald G (eds) *Quality, Evidence and Effectiveness in Health Promotion.* Routledge, London, p. 5–18.

MacDonald T (1998) *Re-thinking Health Promotion.* Routledge, London

Macias W, Stravchansky Lewis L and Smith TL (2005) Health-related message boards/chat rooms on the web: Discussion content and implications for pharmaceutical sponsorships. *Journal of Health Communication* 10 (3): 209–223.

Magnoc D, Tomaka J and Bridges-Arzaga A (2011) Using the web to increase physical activity in college students. *American Journal of Health Behaviour* 35 (2): 142–154.

Marek E, Dergez T, Bozsa S, Gocze K, Rebek - Nagy G, Kricskovics A, Kiss I, Ember I, Gocze P (2011) Incomplete knowledge – unclarified roles in sex education: results of a national survey about human papillomavirus infections. *European Journal of Cancer Care* 20 (6) 759–768.

Markens S, Fox SA, Taub B and Gilbert ML (2002) Role of black churches in health promotion programs: Lessons from the Los Angeles mammography promotion in churches program. *American Journal of Public Health* 92 (5): 805–810.

Marks L (2003) Evidence-based practice in tackling inequalities in health. Report of a research and development project, University of Durham; available at www.dur.ac.uk/resources/public.health/publications/Inequalities%20Report.pdf, last accessed 20 April 2012.

Marr B and Kershaw J (1998) *Caring for older people. Developing specialist practice.* Hodder Arnold, London.

Marston C (2004) Gendered communication among young people in Mexico: Implications for sexual health interventions. *Social Science and Medicine* 59 (3): 445–456.

Martinson BE and Hindman DB (2005) Building a health promotion agenda in local newspapers. *Health Education Research* 20 (1): 51–60.

Matthews B (2004) Grey literature: Resources for locating unpublished research. *C&RL News* 65 (3): 518–519.

Mazor KM, Calvi J, Cowan R, Costanza ME, Han PK, Greene SM, Saccoccio L, Cove E and Williams RD (2010) Media messages about cancer: What do people understand? *Journal of Health Communication* 15 (Suppl. 2): 126–145.

McCartney M (2011) The press release, relative risks and the polypill. *British Medical Journal* 343: 4720.

McCormack LA, Laska MN, Larson NI and Story M (2010) Review of the nutritional implications of farmers' markets and community gardens: A call for evaluation and research efforts. *Journal of the American Dietetic Association* 110 (3): 399–408.

McCoy MR, Couch D, Duncan ND and Lynch GS (2005) Evaluating an Internet weight-loss program for diabetes prevention. *Health Promotion International* 20 (3): 221–228.

McDaniel AM, Casper GR, Hutchinson SK and Stratton RM (2005) Design and testing of an interactive smoking cessation intervention for inner-city women. *Health Education Research* 20 (3): 379–384.

McQueen DV (2000) Strengthening the evidence base for health promotion. *Health Promotion International* 16 (3): 261–268.

McQueen DV (2002) The evidence debate (editorial). *Journal of Epidemiology and Community Health* 56 (2): 83–84.

Mejia-Downs A, Fruth SJ, Clifford A, Hine S, Huckstep J, Wilkinson H and Yoder J (2011) A preliminary exploration of the effects of a 6-week interactive video dance exercise program in an adult population. *Cardiopulmonary Physical Therapy Journal* 22 (4): 5–11.

Mencap (2012) *Stand By Me*; available at www.mencap.org.uk/standbyme, last accessed 16 November 2012.

Mevissen FEF, Ruiter RAC, Meertens RM, Zimbile F and Schaalma HP (2011) Justify your love: Testing an online STI risk communication intervention designed to promote condom use and STI testing. *Psychology and Health* 26 (2): 205–221.

Mier N, Ory MG and Medina AA (2010) Anatomy of culturally sensitive interventions promoting nutrition and exercise in Hispanics: A critical examination of existing literature. *Health Promotion Practice* 11 (4): 541–554.

Milton K, Kelly P, Bull F and Foster CA (2011) Formative evaluation of a family-based walking intervention – Furness Families Walk4 Life. *BMC Public Health* 11: 614.

Minardi H and Riley M (1997) *Communication in Health Care: A skills-based approach.* Butterworth-Heinemann, London.

Monahan JL (1995) Thinking positively using positive affect when designing health messages, pp. 81–98 in Maibach E and Parrott RL (eds) *Designing Health Messages.* Sage, London.

Moodi M, Mood MB, Sharifirad GR, Shahnazi H and Sharifzadeh G (2011) Evaluation of breast self examination program using health belief model in female students. *Journal of Research in Medical Science* 16 (3): 316–322.

Mooney A, Statham J, Boddy J and Smith M (2010) The National Child Measurement Programme: Early experiences of routine feedback to parents of children's weight and height. Institute of Education, University of London; available at www.change4lifewm.org.uk/resources/temp_-_early_experiences_of_routine_feedback.pdf, last accessed 20 April 2012.

Moorley CR (2012) Life after stroke: Personal, social and cultural factors – an inner city Afro Caribbean experience. PhD thesis, University of East London.

MORI (2005) Technology tracker. Technology research information, MORI; available at www.ipsos-mori.com, last accessed 16 November 2012.

Morrell P (2001) Social factors affecting communication, pp. 33–44 in Ellis RB, Gates RJ and Kenworthy N (eds) *Interpersonal Communication in Nursing.* Churchill Livingstone, London.

Moser RP, Green V, Weber D and Doyle C (2005) Psychosocial correlates of fruit and vegetable consumption among African American men. *Journal of Nutrition Education and Behaviour* 37 (6): 306–314.

Murnaghan DA, Blanchard CM, Rodgers WM, LaRosa JN, MacQuarrie CR, MacLellan DL and Gray BJ (2010) Predictors of physical activity, healthy eating and being smoke-free in teens: A theory of planned behaviour approach. *Psychology and Health* 25 (8): 925–941.

Muturi N and An S (2010) HIV/AIDS stigma and religiosity among African American women. *Journal of Health Communication* 15 (4): 388–401.

Naidoo J and Wills J (2009) *Public Health and Health Promotion Practice*, 3rd edition. Balliere Tindall, London.

National Cancer Institute (2010) Evaluating online sources of information; available at www.cancer.gov, last accessed 20 April 2012.

NSMC (2011) The big pocket guide available at thensmc.com/sites/default/files/Big_pocket_guide_2011.pdf, last accessed 20 August 2012 .

Nayak S, Roberts MS, Chang CH and Greenspan SL (2010) Health beliefs about osteoporosis and osteoporosis screening in older women and men. *Health Education Journal* 69 (3): 267–276.

Neale J, McKeganey N, Hay G and Oliver J (2001) Recreational drug use and driving: A qualitative study. The Scottish Executive Central Research Unit, The Stationery Office, Edinburgh; available at www.scotland.gov.uk.

Netto G, Bhopal R, Lederle N, Khatoon J and Jackson A (2010) How can health promotion interventions be adapted for minority ethnic communities? Five principles for guiding the development of behaviour interventions. *Health Promotion International* 25 (2): 248–57.

Neuhauser L and Kreps GL (2008) Online cancer communication: Meeting the literacy, cultural and linguistic needs of diverse audiences. *Patient Education and Counseling* 71 (3): 365–377.

Newman M and Harrier D (2006) Teaching and learning resources for evidence-based practice; available at www.mdx.ac.uk.

NHS Centre for Reviews and Dissemination (2001) Undertaking systematic reviews of research on effectiveness: CRD's guidance for those carrying out or commissioning reviews. *CRD Report 4*, 2nd edn; available at www.york.ac.uk/inst/crd/pdf/Systematic_Reviews.pdf, last accessed 20 April 2012.

NHS Health Scotland (2007) Healthy Living Neighbourhood Shops project: A report on the success of marketing healthy options in convenience stores in Scotland; available at www.healthscotland.com/uploads/documents/3857-Healthyliving_Neighbourhood_Shops_Project.pdf, last accessed 20 April 2012.

NICE (2005) Proposals for making the guideline development process more efficient. Consultation document; available at www.nice.org.uk/niceMedia/pdf/boardmeeting/brdnov05item5b.pdf, last accessed 20 April 2012.

NICE (2008) Guidance for midwives, health visitors, pharmacists and other primary care services to improve the nutrition of pregnant and breastfeeding mothers and children in low income households. Public Health Guidance PH11; available at http://guidance.nice.org.uk/PH11, last accessed 20 April 2012.

NICE (2010) Preventing unintentional injuries in children and young people under 15: Road design and modification self-assessment tool. Public Health Guidance PH31; available at http://guidance.nice.org.uk/PH31, last accessed 20 April 2012.

NICE (2011) Preventing type 2 diabetes: Population and community-level interventions in high-risk groups and the general population. Public Health Guidance PH35; available at http://guidance.nice.org.uk/PH35, last accessed 20 April 2012.

Niederdeppe J, Farrelly MC, Nonnemaker J, Davis KC and Wagner L (2011) Socioeconomic variation in recall and perceived effectiveness of campaign advertisements to promote smoking cessation. *Social Science and Medicine* 72 (5): 773–780.

Noar SM (2006) A 10-year retrospective of research in health mass media campaigns: Where do we go from here? *Journal of Health Communication* 11 (1): 21–42.

Noar SM (2012) An audience-channel-message-evaluation (ACME) framework for health communication campaigns. *Health Promotion Practice* 13 (4): 481–8.

Northouse LL and Northouse PG (1998) *Health Communication: Strategies for health professionals*, 3rd edition. Appleton and Lange, London.

Nutbeam D (1999) The challenge to provide 'evidence' in health promotion (Editorial). *Health Promotion International* 14 (2): 99–101.

O'Donnell MP (2009) Definition of health promotion 2.0: Embracing passion, enhancing motivation, recognising dynamic balance and creating opportunities. *American Journal Health Promotion* 24 (1): iv.

O'Grady L, Wittemann H, Bender JL, Urowitz S, Wiljer D and Jadad AR (2009) Measuring the impact of a moving target: A dynamic framework for evaluating collaborative, adaptive, interactive technologies. *Journal of Medical Internet Research* 11(2): e20.

O'Halloran R, Hickson L and Worrall L (2008) Environmental factors that influence communication between people with communication disability and their healthcare providers in hospital: A review of the literature within the International Classification of Functioning, Disability and Health (ICF) framework. *International Journal of Communication Disorders* 43 (6): 601–632.

O'Hegarty M, Pederson LL, Nelson DF, Mowery P, Gable JM and Wortley P (2006) Reactions of young adult smokers to warning labels on cigarette packages. *American Journal of Preventive Medicine* 30 (6): 467–473.

Office for National Statistics (ONS) (2001) Census 2001; available at www.ons.gov.uk/ons/guide-method/census/census-2001/index.html, last accessed 20 April 2012.

Office for National Statistics (ONS) (2006) Social trends 41 available at www.ons.gov.uk/ons/rel/social.../social-trends-41---e-society.pdf, last accessed 20 August 2012.

Oronje RN, Undie CC, Zulu EM and Crichton J (2011) Engaging media in communicating research on sexual and reproductive health and rights in sub-Saharan Africa: Experiences and lessons learned. *Health Research and Policy Systems* 16 (9, Suppl. 1): S7.

Overseas Development Institute (2006) Evidence-based policy making; available at www.odi.org.uk/resources/details.asp?id=2804&title=evidence-based-policymaking-work-relevance-developing-countries, last accessed 20 April 2012.

Oyediran KA, Feyosetan OI and Akpan T (2011) Predictors of condom-use among young never-married males in Nigeria. *Journal of Health and Population Nutrition* 29 (3): 273–285.

Padilla RP, Bill S, Raghunath SG, Fernald D, Havranek EP and Steiner JF (2010) Designing a cardiovascular disease prevention website for Latinos: Qualitative community feedback. *Health Promotion Practice* 11 (1): 140–147.

Paek H, Hilyard K, Freimuth V, Barge JK and Mindlin M (2010) Theory-based approaches to understanding public emergency preparedness: Implications for effective health and risk communication. *Journal of Health Communication* 15 (4): 428–444.

Panagopoulou E, Montgomery A and Benos A (2011) Health promotion as a behavioural challenge: Are we missing attitudes? *Global Health Promotion* 18 (2): 54–57.

Parker EA, Baldwin GT, Israel B and Salinas M (2004) Application of health promotion theories and models for environmental health. *Health Education and Behaviour* 31 (4): 491–509.

Pechmann C and Reibling ET (2000) Anti-smoking advertising campaigns targeting youth: Case studies from USA and Canada. *Tobacco Control* 9 (Suppl. ii): ii8–ii31.

Peterson J, Atwood JR and Yates B (2002) Key elements for church-based health promotion programs: Outcome-based literature review. *Public Health Nursing* 19 (6): 401–411.

Peterson M, Abraham A and Waterfield A (2005) Marketing physical activity: Lessons learned from a statewide media campaign. *Health Promotion Practice* 6 (4): 437–446.

Philips-Guzman CM, Martinez-Donate AP, Hovell MF, Blumberg EJ, Sipan CL, Rovinak LS and Kelley NJ (2011) Engaging local businesses in HIV prevention efforts: The consumer perspective. *Health Promotion Practice* 12 (4): 620–629.

Phillips RO, Ulleberg P and Vaa T (2011) Meta-analysis of the effect of road safety campaign on accidents. *Accident Analysis and Prevention* 43 (3): 1204–1218.

Plant A, Montoya JA, Rotblatt H, Kerndt PR, Mall KL, Pappas LG, Kent CK and Klausner JD (2010) Stop the sores: The making and evaluation of a successful social marketing campaign. *Health Promotion Practice* 11 (1): 23–33.

Poland B and Dooris M (2010) A green and healthy future: The settings approach to building health, equity and sustainability. *Critical Public Health* 20 (3): 281–298.

Poland B, Krupa G and McCall D (2009) Settings for health promotion: An analytic framework to guide intervention design and implementation. *Health Promotion Practice* 10 (4): 505–516.

Population Communication Services/Center for Communication Programs (JHU/CCP) (2003) A field guide to designing a health communication strategy. Johns Hopkins University; available at www.jhuccp.org/node/1033, last accessed 20 August 2012.

Population Reference Bureau (PRB) (2005) Promoting healthy behaviour; available at www.prb.org/pdf05/promotinghealthybehavior_eng.pdf, last accessed 20 April 2012.

Povlsen L, Olsen B and Ladelund S (2005) Educating families from ethnic minorities in type 1 diabetes: Experiences from a Danish intervention study. *Patient Education and Counseling* 59 (2): 164–170.

Prochaska JO and Diclemente CC (1983) Stages and processes of self-change in smoking: Toward an integrative model of change. *Journal of Consulting and Clinical Psychology* 51 (3): 390–395.

Purdy C (2011) Using the Internet and social media to promote condom use in Turkey. *Reproductive Health Matters* 19 (37): 157–165.

Rada J, Ratima M and Howden-Chapman P (1999) Evidence-based purchasing of health promotion: Methodology for reviewing evidence. *Health Promotion International* 14 (2): 177–187.

Randolf W and Viswanath K (2004) Lessons learned from public health mass media campaigns: marketing health in a crowded media world. *Annual Review of Public Health* 25 (1): 419–437.

Raphael D (2000) The question of evidence in health promotion. *Health Promotion International* 15 (4): 355–367.

Reid LV, Hatch J and Parrish T (2003) The role of a historically black university and the black church in community-based health initiatives: The project DIRECT experience. *Journal of Public Health Management Practice* November (Suppl.): S70–73.

Reinert B, Campbell C, Carver V and Range LM (2003) Joys and tribulations of faith-based youth tobacco prevention: a case study in Mississippi. *Health Education Practice* 4 (3): 228–238.

Reinert B, Carver V, Range LM and Pike C (2008) Collecting health data with youth at faith-based institutions: Lessons learned. *Health Promotion Practice* 9 (1): 68–73.

Reininger BM, Barroso CS, Mitchell Bennett L, Cantu E, Fernandez ME, Gonzalez DA, Chavez M, Freeberg D and McAllister AL (2010) Process evaluation and participatory methods in an obesity prevention media campaign for Mexican Americans. *Health Promotion Practice* 11 (3): 347–357.

Releford BJ, Frencher SK and Yancey AK (2010a) Health promotion in barbershops: Balancing outreach and research in African American communities. *Ethnicity and Diversity* 20 (2): 185–188.

Releford BJ, Frencher SK, Yancey AK and Norris K (2010b) Cardiovascular disease control through barbershops: Design of a nationwide outreach program. *Journal of the National Medical Association* 102 (4): 336–345.

Resnicow K, Jackson A, Braithwaite R, DiIorio C, Blisset D, Rahotep S and Periasamy S (2002) Health body/health spirit: A church-based nutrition and physical activity intervention. *Health Education Research* 17 (5): 562–573.

Resnicow K, Jackson A, Wang T, De AK, McCarty F, Dudley W and Baranowski T (2001) A motivational interviewing intervention to increase fruit and vegetable intake through black churches: Results of the eat for life trial. *American Journal of Public Health* 91 (10): 1686–1693.

Ribisl KM (2003) The potential of the Internet as a medium to encourage and discourage youth tobacco use. *Tobacco Control* 12 (Suppl. 1): i48–i59.

Rice D (2001) The internet and health communication: a framework of experiences, pp. 5–46 in Rice RE and Katz JE (eds) *The Internet and health communication: experiences and expectations*. London: Sage.

Rimal RN and Lapinski MK (2009) Why health communication is important in public health. *Bulletin World Health Organization* 87 (4): 247–248.

Risi L, Bindman JP, Campbell OMR, Imrie J, Everett K, Bradley J and Denny L (2004) Media interventions to increase cervical screening uptake in South Africa: An evaluation of effectiveness. *Health Education Research* 19 (4): 457–468.

Robinson L (2004) Beliefs, values and intercultural communication, pp. 110–120 in Robb M, Barrett S, Komaromy C and Rogers A (eds) *Communication, Relationships and Care: A reader*. Routledge, London.

Robinson M (2002) *Communication and Health in a Multi-ethnic Society*. Policy Press, Bristol.

Roelens K, Verstraelen H, Van Egmond K and Temmerman M (2006) A knowledge, attitudes, and practice survey among obstetrician-gynaecologists on intimate partner violence in Flanders, Belgium. *BMC Public Health* 6: 238.

Romer D, Sznitman S, DiClemente R, Salazar LF, Vanable PA, Carey MP, Hennessy M, Brown LK, Valois RF, Stanton BF, Fortune T and Juzang I (2009) Mass media as an HIV prevention strategy: Using culturally sensitive messages to reduce HIV associated sexual behaviour of at risk African American youth. *American Journal of Public Health* 99 (12): 2150–2159.

Rosenstock IM (1966) Why people use health services. *Milbank Memorial Fund Quarterly* XLIV 3 (2): 94–127.

Rosenstock IM, Stretcher VJ and Becker MM (1988) Social learning theory and the health belief model. *Health Education Quarterly* 15 (2): 175–183.

Rossi PH, Lipsey MW and Freeman HE (2004) *Evaluation: A systematic approach*, 7th edition. Sage, Thousand Oaks, CA.

Rowe R and Garcia J (2003) Evidence on access to maternity and infant care in England. National Perinatal Epidemiological Unit, Oxford.

Russell CA, Clapp JD and DeJong W (2005) Done 4: Analysis of a failed social norms marketing campaign. *Health Communication* 17 (1): 57–65.

Rutter D and Quine L (eds) (2002) *Changing Health Behaviour*. Open University Press, Buckingham.

Ruud JS, Betts N, Kritch K, Nitzke S, Lohse B and Boeckner L (2005) Acceptability of stage-tailored newsletters about fruit and vegetables by young adults. *Journal of the American Dietetic Association* 105 (11): 1774–1778.

Rychetnik L and Wise M (2004) Advocating evidence-based health promotion: Reflections and a way forward. *Health Promotion International* 19 (2): 247–257.

Sackett D, Rosenberg W, Muir Grey JAM, Hayes RB and Williamson WS (1996) Evidence-based medicine: What it is and what it isn't (editorial). *British Medical Journal* 312: 71–72.

Salehi L, Mohammad K and Montazeri A (2011) Fruit and vegetables intake among elderly Iranians: A theory-based interventional study using the five-a-day program. *Nutrition Journal* 14 (10): 123.

Samaritans, The (2006) txt Samaritans 4 emotional support; available at www.samaritans. org.uk.

Scheier LM and Grenard JL (2010) Influence of a nationwide social marketing campaign on adolescent drug use. *Journal of Health Communication* 15 (3): 240–271.

Schüza B, Marx C, Wurm S, Warner C, Ziegelmann JP, Schwarzer R and Tesch-Römera C (2011) Medication beliefs predict medication adherence in older adults. *Journal of Psychosomatic Research* 70 (2): 179–187.

Sebastian MP, Khan ME and Roychowdhury S (2010) Promoting healthy spacing between pregnancies in India: Need for differential education campaigns. *Patient Education and Counseling* 81 (3): 395–401.

Shafer A, Cates JR, Diehl SJ and Hartmann M (2011) Asking Mom: Formative research for an HPV vaccine campaign targeting mothers of adolescent girls. *Journal of Health Communication* 16 (9): 988–1005.

Sharangpani R, Boulton KE, Wells E and Kim C (2011) Attitudes and behaviours of international air travellers toward pandemic influenza. *Journal of Travel Medicine* 18 (3): 203–208.

Sharp C (2005) The improvement of public sector delivery: Supporting evidence-based practice through action research. September, Scottish Executive Research; available at www. scotland.gov.uk/Publications/2005.

Sivaram S, Johnson S, Bentley ME, Go VF, Lakin C, Srikishnam AK, Celentono K and Solomon S (2005) Sexual health promotion in Chennai, India: The key role of communication among social networks. *Health Promotion International* 20 (4): 327–333.

Smith BJ, Tang KC and Nutbeam D (2006) WHO health promotion glossary: New terms. *Health Promotion International* 20 (1): 1–6.

Solomon FM, Linnan LA, Wasilewski Y, Lee AM, Katz MI and Yang J (2004) Observational study in ten beauty salons: Results informing development of the North Carolina BEAUTY and health project. *Health Education and Behaviour* 31 (6): 790–807.

Sowden AJ and Arblaster L (2006) Mass media interventions for preventing smoking in young people (Review). *The Cochrane Library* Issue 1; available at http://onlinelibrary. wiley.com/doi/10.1002/14651858.CD001006/pdf/standard, last accessed 20 April 2012.

Sparks L and Nussbaum JF (2008) Health literacy and cancer communication with older adults. *Patient Education and Counseling* 71 (3): 345–350.

Spear Z (2009) Pinch media: iPhone app usage declining rapidly after first downloads; available at www.appleinsider.com/articles/09/02/19/iphone_app_usage_declining_rapidly_ after_first_downloads.html, last accessed 20 April 2012.

Speller V, Wimbush E and Morgan A (2005) Evidence-based health promotion practice: How to make it work. *Global Health Promotion* 12 (Suppl. 1): 15–20.

Spotswood F and Tapp A (2010) Socio cultural change – the key to social marketing success? A case study of increasing exercise in working class communities. *International Journal of Health Promotion and Education* 48 (2): 52–57.

Sridharan S and Nakaima A (2011) Ten steps to making evaluation matter. *Evaluation and Program Planning* 34 (2): 135–146.

Stephenson CM and Stephenson MR (2011) Hearing loss prevention for carpenters: part 1: Using health communication and health promotion models to develop training that works. *Noise Health* 13: 113–121.

Strandbygaard U, Thomsen SF and Backer V (2010) A daily reminder increases adherence to asthma treatment: A three-month follow-up study. *Respiratory Medicine* 104 (2): 166–171.

Stretcher VJ, Shiffman S and West R (2005) Randomised controlled trial of a web-based computer-tailored smoking cessation program as a supplement to nicotine patch therapy. *Addiction* 100 (5): 682–688.

Sugerman S, Backman D, Foester SB, Ghirardelli A, Linares A and Fong A (2011) Using an opinion poll to build an obesity prevention social marketing campaign for low income Asian and Hispanic immigrants: Report of findings. *Journal of Nutrition Education and Behaviour* 43 (4, Suppl. 2): S53–S66.

Suggs LS (2006) A 10-year retrospective of research in new technologies for health communication. *Journal of Health Communication* 11 (1): 61–74.

Suresh K (2011) Evidence-based communication for health promotion: Indian lessons of the last decade. *Public Health Education* 55 (4): 276–285.

Swinney J, Anson-Wonkka C, Maki E and Corneau J (2001) Community assessment: A church community and the parish nurse. *Public Health Nursing* 18 (1): 40–44.

Synder L (2007) Health communication campaigns and their impact on behaviour. *Journal of Nutrition Education and Behaviour* 39 (2, Suppl.): S32–S40.

Talk to Frank (2012) *Talk to Frank*; available at www.talktofrank.com/, last accessed 16 November 2012.

Tang KC, Ehsani JP and McQueen DV (2003) Evidence-based health promotion: Recollections, reflections and reconsiderations. *Journal of Epidemiology and Community Health* 57 (11): 841–843.

Taylor M, Dlamini SB, Meyer-Weitz A, Sathipardsad R, Jinabhai CC and Esterhuizen Y (2010) Changing sexual behaviour to reduce HIV transmission – a multi-faceted approach to HIV prevention and treatment in a rural South Africa setting. *AIDS Care* 22 (11): 1395–1402.

Taylor-Clarke KA, Viswanath K and Blendon RJ (2010) Communication inequalities during public health disasters: Katrina's wake. *Health Communication* 25 (3): 221–229.

TeHIP (2005) The impact of e-health and assistive technologies in health care. The E-health Innovation Professionals Group; available at www.tehip.org.uk, last accessed 20 April 2012.

Text4Baby (2012) www.text4baby.org, last accessed 20 April 2012.

Thackeray R and Neiger BL (2009) A multidirectional communication model: Implications for social marketing practice. *Health Promotion Practice* 10 (2): 171–175.

Thackeray R, Keller H, Heilbronner JM and Dellinger LK (2011) Social marketing's unique contribution to mental health stigma reduction and HIV testing: Two case studies. *Health Promotion Practice* 12 (2): 172–177.

Thalacker KM (2011) Hypertension and the Hmong community: Using the health belief model for health promotion. *Health Promotion Practice* 12 (4): 538–543.

Thesenvitz J, Hershfield L and Macdonald R (2011) Health communication outcomes: At the heart of good objectives and indicators. Public Health Ontario; available at www.thcu.ca/resource_db/pubs/898209026.pdf, last accessed 20 April 2012.

Thompson CA and Ravia J (2011) A systematic review of behavioural interventions to promote intake of fruit and vegetables. *Journal of the American Dietetic Association* 111 (10): 1523–1535.

Thompson L and Kumar A (2011) Responses to health promotion campaigns: Resistance, denial and othering. *Critical Public Health* 21 (1): 105–117.

Thompson N (2002) *People Skills*, 2nd edition. Palgrave Macmillan, Basingstoke.

Thorogood M and Coombes Y (eds) (2010) *Evaluating Health Promotion: Practice and methods*, 2nd edition. Oxford University Press, Oxford.

Thurston WE and Blundell-Gosselin HJ (2005) The farm as a setting for health promotion: Results of a needs assessment in South Central Alberta. *Health and Place* 11 (1): 31–43.

Tinker A (1997) *Older People in Modern Society.* Longman, London.

Tolvanen M, Lahti S, Miettunen J and Hausen H (2011) Relationship between oral health-related knowledge, attitudes and behaviour among 15–16-year-old adolescents – A structural equation modelling approach. *Acta Odontologica Scandinavica* 70 (2): 169–176.

Tomassini C (2005) The demographic characteristics of the oldest old in the United Kingdom. *Population Trends* 120 (Summer): 15–22.

Tones K and Tilford S (1994) *Health Education: Effectiveness, efficiency and equity*, 2nd edition. Chapman and Hall, London.

Trifiletti LB, Gielen AC, Sleet DA and Hopkins K (2005) Behavioural and social sciences theories and models: Are they used in unintentional injury prevention research? *Health Education Research* 20 (3): 298–307.

Tsouros AD, Dowding G, Thompson J and Dooris M (eds) (1998) Health promoting universities, concept experience and framework for action. WHO, Copenhagen; available at www.who.dk/document/E60163.pdf, last accessed 20 April 2012.

Turner-McGrievy G and Tate D (2011) Tweets, apps, and pods: Results of the 6 month mobile pounds off digitally (Mobile POD) randomised weight-loss intervention among adults. *Journal of Medical Internet Research* 13 (4): e120.

Twomby EC, Holtz KD and Tessman GK (2008) Multimedia science education on drugs of abuse: A preliminary evaluation of effectiveness for adolescents. Letter to the editor. *Journal of Alcohol and Drug Education* 55 (1): 8.

University of Central Lancashire (UCLAN) (2006) Health settings development unit; available at www.uclan.ac.uk/facs/health/hsdu/index.htm, last accessed 20 April 2012.

Unni EJ and Farris KB (2011) Unintentional non adherence and belief in medicine in older adults. *Patient Education and Counseling* 83 (2): 265–268.

US Department of Health and Human Services (2010) Healthy people 2020 brochure available at www.healthypeople.gov/2020/TopicsObjectives2020/pdfs/HP2020_brochure_with_LHI_508.pdf

US Office of Disease Prevention and Health Promotion (2010) Healthy people 2020; available at www.healthypeople.gov/document, last accessed 20 April 2012.

Vallone DM, Duke JC, Cullen J, McCausland KL and Allen JA (2011) Evaluation of EX: A national mass media smoking cessation campaign. *American Journal of Public Health* 101 (2): 302–309.

Van Cauwenberghe E, Maes L, Spittaels H, Van Lenthe FJ, Brug J, Oppert JM and De Bourdeaudhuij I (2010) Effectiveness of school-based interventions in Europe to promote healthy nutrition in children and adolescents: Systematic review of published and 'grey' literature. *British Journal of Nutrition* 103 (6): 781–797.

Van den Putte B, Yzer M, Southwell BG, de Bruijin GJ and Willemsen MC (2011) Interpersonal communication as an indirect pathway for the effect of antismoking media content on smoking cessation. *Journal of Health Communication* 16 (5): 470–485.

Van Gemert C, Dietze P, Gold J, Sacks-Davis R, Stoove M, Vally H and Hellard M (2011) The Australian National Binge Drinking campaign: Campaign recognition among young people at the music festival who report risky drinking. *BMC Public Health* 20 (11): 482.

Viswanath K and Ackerson LK (2011) Race, ethnicity, language, social class, and health communication inequalities: A nationally-representative cross sectional study. *PloS One* 6 (1): e14550.

Vydelingum V (2000) South Asian patients' lived experience of acute care in an English hospital. *Journal of Advanced Nursing* 32 (1): 100–107.

Wakefield MA, Loken B and Hornik RC (2010) Use of mass media campaigns to change health behaviour. *The Lancet* 376: 1261–1271.

Wallace S (1998) Telemedicine in the NHS for the millennium and beyond, pp. 55–99 in Lenaghan J (ed.) *Rethinking IT and Health*. Institute for Public Policy Research. London.

Wallcraft J (2003) *The Mental Health Service User Movement in England*. Sainsbury Centre for Mental Health, London.

Walsh M, Cartwright L, Cornish C, Sugrue S and Wood-Martin R (2011) The body composition, nutritional knowledge, attitudes, behaviours and future education needs of senior schoolboy rugby players in Ireland. *International Journal of Sport, Nutrition and Exercise Metabolism* 21 (5): 365–376.

Wang G and Labarthe D (2011) The cost effectiveness of interventions designed to reduce sodium intake. *Journal of Hypertension* 29 (9): 1693–1699.

Wang M, Macdonald VM, Paudel M and Banke KK (2011) National scale up of zinc promotion in Nepal: Results from a post-project population-based survey. *Journal of Health Nutrition* 29 (3): 207–217.

Wang S, Moss JR and Hiller JE (2005) Applicability and transferability of interventions in evidence-based public health. *Health Promotion International* 21 (1): 76–83.

Wanyoni KL, Themessl-Huber M, Humphries G and Freeman R (2011) A systematic review and meta-analysis of face-to-face communication of tailored health messages: Implications for practice. *Patient Education and Counseling* 85 (3): 348–355.

Watzlawick P, Beavin J and Jackson D (1967) *The Pragmatics of Human Communication*. Norton, New York.

Webb OJ, Eves FF and Kerr J (2011) A statistical summary of mall-based stair-climbing interventions. *Journal Physical Activity and Health* 8 (4): 558–565.

Weinberg DS, Turner BJ, Wang H, Myers RE and Miller S (2004) A survey of women regarding factors affecting colorectal cancer screening compliance. *Preventive Medicine* 38 (6): 669–675.

Weinreich NK (2011) *Hands-on Social Marketing*. Sage, London.

Weitkunat R, Pottgiesser C, Meyer N, Crispin A, Fischer R, Scotten K, Keir J and Überla K (2003) Perceived risk of bovine spongiform encephalopathy and dietary behaviour. *Journal of Health Psychology* 8 (3): 373–381.

West R (2005) Time for a change: Putting the transtheoretical model to rest. (Editorial). *Addiction* 11 (8): 1036–1039.

Whitehead D (2004) The health promoting university (HPU): The role and function of nursing. *Nurse Education Today* 24 (6): 466–472.

Whitelaw S, Baxendale A, Bryce C, Machardy L, Young I and Witney E (2001) 'Settings'-based health promotion: A review. *Health Promotion International* 16 (4): 339–353.

Whitelaw S, Graham N, Black D, Coburn J and Renwick L (2012) Developing capacity and achieving sustainable implementation in healthy 'settings': Insights from NHS Health Scotland's Health Promoting Health Service project. *Health Promotion International* 27 (1): 127–137.

Wiggers J and Sanson-Fisher R (2001) Evidence-based health promotion, pp. 126–145 in Scott D and Weston R (eds) *Evaluating Health Promotion*. Nelson Thornes, Cheltenham.

Wilkins A and Mak DB (2007) Sending out an SMSL: An impact and outcome evaluation of the Western Australian Department of Health's 2005 chlamydia campaign. *Health Promotion Journal of Australia* 18 (2): 113–120.

Williams J (2011) The effect on young people of suicide reports in the media. *Mental Health Practice* 14 (8): 34–37.

Williams M, Bowen A and Ei S (2010) An evaluation of the experiences of rural MSM who accessed an online HIV/AIDS health promotion intervention. *Health Promotion Practice* 11 (4): 474–482.

Wilson BJ (2007) Designing media messages about health and nutrition: What strategies are the most effective? *Journal of Nutrition Education and Behaviour* 39 (2, Suppl.): S13–S19.

Witte K (2007) Theory-based interventions and evaluations of outreach efforts. National Network of Libraries for Medicine; available at www.nnlm.gov/evaluation/pub/witte, last accessed 20 April 2012.

Wong C and Tang CS (2005) Practice of habitual and volitional health behaviours to prevent severe acute respiratory syndrome among Chinese adolescents in Hong Kong. *Journal of Adolescent Health* 36 (3): 193–200.

Wong LP and Sam I (2010) Public sources of information and information needs for pandemic influenza A (H1N1). *Journal of Community Health* 35 (6): 676–682.

World Bank (2012) Disabilities; available at http://youthink.worldbank.org/issues/disabilities, last accessed 20 April 2012.

World Health Assembly (WHA) (1998) Resolution WHA 51.12 on health promotion: agenda item 20. WHO 16 May; available at www.who.int, last accessed 20 April 2012.

World Health Organization (WHO) (1986) Ottawa Charter for Health Promotion, 17–21 November, Ottawa; available at www.who.int/hpr/NPH/docs/ottawa_charter_hp.pdf, last accessed 20 April 2012.

World Health Organization (WHO) (1998) Health promotion: Milestones on the road to a global alliance. Fact sheet No. 171 revised June 1998; available at www.who.int, last accessed 20 April 2012.

World Health Organization (WHO) (2000) International classification of impairments, disabilities and handicaps. WHO, Geneva; available at www.who.int, last accessed 20 April 2012.

World Health Organization (WHO) (2003) Healthy cities around the world: An overview of the healthy cities movement in six WHO regions. WHO, Belfast; available at www.euro.who.int/document/hcp/healthycityworld.pdf, last accessed 20 April 2012.

Wright E, Fortune T, Juzang I and Bull S (2011) Text messaging for HIV prevention with young black men: Formative research and campaign development. *AIDS Care* 23 (5): 534–541.

Xiangyang T, Lan Z, Xueping M, Tao Z, Yuzhen S and Jagusztyn M (2003) Beijing health promoting universities: Practice and evaluation. *Health Promotion International* 18 (2): 107–113.

Yao CS, Merz EL, Nakaji M, Harry KM, Malcarne VL and Sadler GR (2012) Cervical cancer control: Deaf and hearing women's response to an educational video. *Journal of Cancer Education* 27 (1): 62–66.

Yorkston KM, Bourgeois MS and Baylor CR (2010) Communication and aging. *Physical Medical and Rehabilitation Clinics of North America* 21 (2): 309–319.

Zaidi SM, Bikak AL, Shaheryar A, Imam SH and Khan JA (2011) Perceptions of anti-smoking messages amongst high school students in Pakistan. *BMC Public Health* 18 (11): 117.

Zazove P, Meador HE, Reed BD, Sen A and Gorenflo DW (2012) Effectiveness of videos improving cancer prevention knowledge in people with profound hearing loss. *Journal of Cancer Education* 12 April [Epub ahead of publication].

Zondervan M, Kuper H, Solomon A and Buchan J (2004) Health promotion for trachoma control. *Community Eye Health Journal* 17 (52): 57–58.

Zuure FR, Davidovich U, Coutinho RA, Kok G, Hoebe CJ, Van den Hoek A, Jansen PL, Van Leeuwen-Gilbert P, Verheuvel NC, Weegink CJ and Prins M (2011) Using mass media and the internet as tools to diagnose hepatitis C infections in the general population. *American Journal of Preventive Medicine* 40 (3): 345–352.

INDEX